Reading by Moonlight

ALSO BY BRENDA WALKER

Crush

One More River

Poe's Cat

The Wing of Night

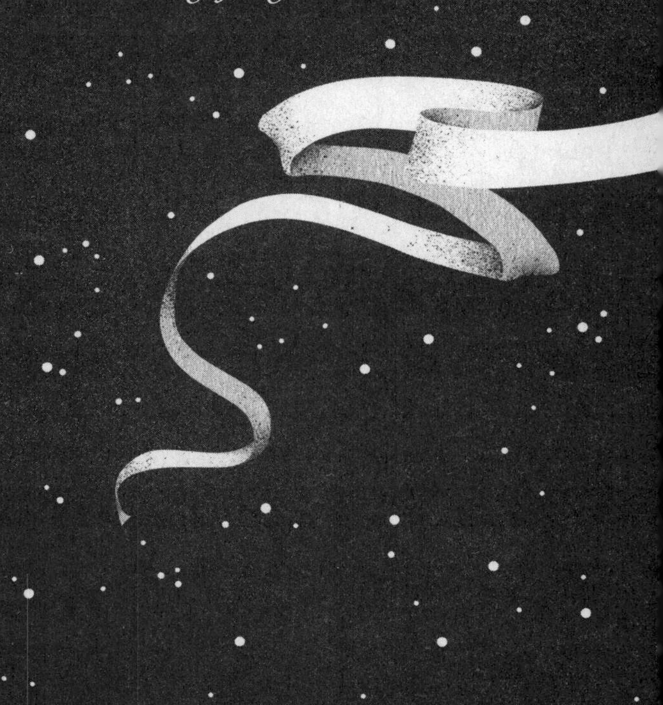

BRENDA WALKER

Reading by Moonlight

How books saved a life

PENGUIN BOOKS

PENGUIN BOOKS

Published by the Penguin Group
Penguin Group (Australia)
250 Camberwell Road, Camberwell, Victoria 3124, Australia
(a division of Pearson Australia Group Pty Ltd)
Penguin Group (USA) Inc.
375 Hudson Street, New York, New York 10014, USA
Penguin Group (Canada)
90 Eglinton Avenue East, Suite 700, Toronto, Canada ON M4P 2Y3
(a division of Pearson Penguin Canada Inc.)
Penguin Books Ltd
80 Strand, London WC2R 0RL, England
Penguin Ireland
25 St Stephen's Green, Dublin 2, Ireland
(a division of Penguin Books Ltd)
Penguin Books India Pvt Ltd
11 Community Centre, Panchsheel Park, New Delhi – 110 017, India
Penguin Group (NZ)
67 Apollo Drive, Rosedale, North Shore 0632, New Zealand
(a division of Pearson New Zealand Ltd)
Penguin Books (South Africa) (Pty) Ltd
24 Sturdee Avenue, Rosebank, Johannesburg 2196, South Africa

Penguin Books Ltd, Registered Offices: 80 Strand, London, WC2R 0RL, England

First published by Penguin Group (Australia), 2010
This paperback edition published 2011

10 9 8 7 6 5 4 3 2 1

Cover design & artwork by Allison Colpoys © Penguin Group (Australia)
Text design by Anne-Marie Reeves & Allison Colpoys © Penguin Group (Australia)
Typeset in Adobe Garamond 12/18 pt by Sunset Digital, Brisbane, Queensland
Printed and bound in Australia by McPherson's Printing Group, Maryborough, Victoria

National Library of Australia
Cataloguing-in-Publication data:

Walker, Brenda, 1957–
Reading by moonlight: how books saved a life/Brenda Walker
9780143205227 (pbk.)
Walker, Brenda, 1957–. Authors, Australian – Biography. Bibliotherapy.

A823.3

penguin.com.au

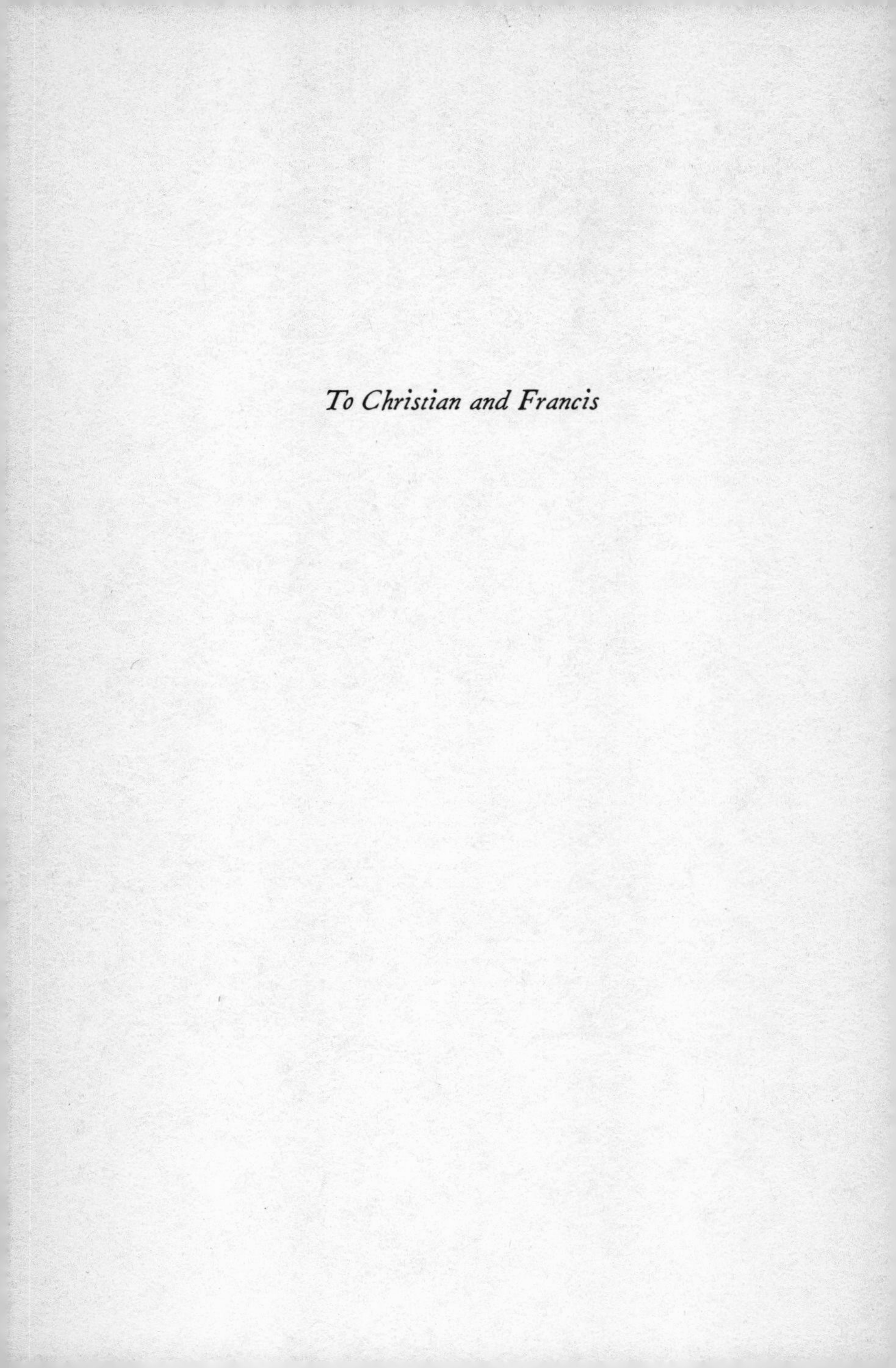

To Christian and Francis

Can the shape of the healing
possibly fit the size of the wound?

JAMES WOOD

CONTENTS

When I was a child my family knew a man with so many books they seemed to push his bed into a corner. They lined the walls from floor to ceiling, and more lay horizontally on those already shelved. Their spines were brushstrokes of ochre and faded orange, violet, red and black. There were even fat chimneys of books rising in the centre of his room.

My own room has sandstone walls and a wooden floor, French doors that open into the upper branches of a Japanese maple which is bare in winter, a mass of green in summer. Birds perch there, tilting their heads to look in at the strange cave where I sleep and work. A few streets away, on the other side of a railway line, there's a long stretch of beach. On cold nights when the waves are high I lie awake to listen to the ocean. There isn't a lot of furniture: a bed, a cupboard, a long white table, and bookshelves with a changing population of spines, because I'm not a collector, I like to hand books on.

Right now my things are bundled into an open bag. Ballet flats, stockings, nightclothes. I'm dressed in jeans and boots and a cotton shirt – my travelling clothes. A friend's car is in the driveway, and as she goes downstairs she calls back to remind me, as if I need reminding, to pack a book.

Hanging above the bed of my parents' friend was a watercolour of a sleeping girl. She lay under a coverlet, her loose hair feathering over pillowy linen. The painting was framed plainly, in dark wood surrounding ordinary reflective glass in which I could see a window and the spines of all those books. The girl seemed to be floating in a transparent library. It suited her, as if pale girls were best seen through the reflection of ink and paper. Looking at the watercolour, I wanted to pull the elastic from my ponytail, free my own hair. Then I looked more closely: the girl's nostrils were plugged for burial.

I was ten or twelve years old at the time, and reading was almost all I did. I skipped sleep, I ducked out of sport at school; it was going to take more than a dead girl to put me off my books. I hadn't read Edgar Allan Poe then; I didn't know that if you were a woman you won a place in a whole poetic tradition by being young, beautiful and dead. But even as a child I knew that although the best books might brush up against sex and death, they're nothing like the real things.

The front door opens downstairs and I haven't moved. I need to think about the book I'm going to put on top of my clothing, my documents, and other necessary things. The book will be the first thing I put my hand on when I arrive, when I'm taken to an empty room in an almost unimaginable place.

I consider taking *The Hours*, by Michael Cunningham. I like the part where Clarissa is wandering through her neighbourhood in New York, shopping for flowers for a party which won't, in the end, take place, although the invitations, the food, the flowers – all the results of her efforts – are close to perfect. She runs into a novelist whose work she doesn't much respect. Clarissa isn't a scornful person; she tries to feel kindly toward this well-meaning and limited man, whose lover is ill.

Later, at a bookshop window, she thinks about buying a gift for the sick man. She doesn't know him very well but she's an editor, she knows about books and she knows exactly what he needs: 'You want to give him the book of his own life, the book that will locate him, parent him, arm him for the changes.' Locate, parent, arm – is it possible? It seems like a lot to ask, but yes, I agree, it's close to what we might hope for from the right book. Of course, Clarissa can't find it, not that day at least, in the window of her local bookshop.

My friend Lauren's voice is coming from the driveway. 'I'll go without you!'

An empty threat. Where would she go? She's here to drive me, to spare me the wait for a taxi, which in this city can arrive immediately, or not at all, or just in time to get you to the check-in desk after the final boarding call. And her car is much better than a taxi, much more comfortable, with her music playing and a statuette of St Rita, patroness of hopeless causes, stuck to the dashboard. We're going to need Rita's help. Parking is always tight at the hospital.

This is the story of the right book, or books. We each have one life, one share of action and vision and money; a single life for all our speech and thought, our decent gestures and the decisions that might undo us, our welcome or unwanted love, our parties that may or may not come off. One life to satisfy our vast and human sense of voyaging. With the right books we find out what imaginary strangers have done with their share of this amazing thing, life.

I'm standing at a bookshop window in my mind. I've chosen some titles for you, the reader. We don't know each other, but I imagine that one day you too might hesitate before you close your carry-bag. There's a book-sized space just under the zip. I hope you're going somewhere beautiful, Ubud, or Kyoto, I may have just the thing. Think of me as a woman who has put a few books to the test.

The story of the books is also the story of the test. It begins with a moment of happiness, and while you can't have a story without a sense of expectancy, without an edge where the known world ends, I try to remind myself that when we leave our rooms and walk to that edge with our eyes closed, we sometimes step from an invisible kerb to a wide, sweet, empty road.

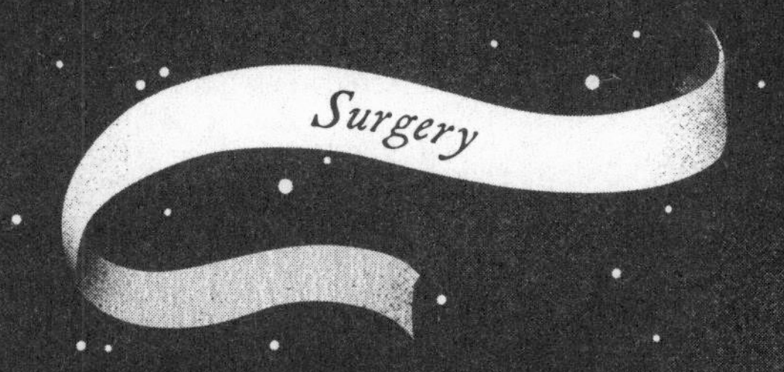
Surgery

It's that time of light excitement just before Christmas when strangers carrying ribboned parcels smile and speak on the street. I'm standing on a footpath in Cottesloe with a bundle of peonies in my arms, sweet as a new baby and almost as heavy. A man stops mid-stride and says, 'You must have been very good.' He thinks the flowers are a gift from a lover. Or he'd like to raise that possibility.

Flowers, love, a quick remark in the street – it comes as a surprise, that sudden, unexpected crackle of flirtation, like the tinsel in the shop windows. I look down at the peonies, skin-pink in my arms. They look like small breasts floating on stems.

'No,' I say, 'they're not mine. They're for a man. And he *was* very good.'

I'm on my way to my reserved and purposeful surgeon. I think he'll like them. He's a breast surgeon. There, I've almost said it. My surgeon has a sign on his door: DISEASES OF THE BREAST.

There are times when I can think of nothing but the moment of my diagnosis, the vertigo as I listened to my GP's explanations: a sense of falling coexisting with a sense of being crushed.

Four years have passed since that diagnosis. Breast cancer: I'm tired of the subject, and I haven't really begun to talk about it yet. To be honest, I'd rather tell you about books. A good book laces invisible fingers into the shape of a winter armchair or a hammock in the sun. I'm not talking about comfort, necessarily, but support. A good writer might take you to strange and difficult places, but you're in the hands of someone you trust.

Yet the books and the illness are deeply involved with each other. We don't leave our bodies behind when we pick up a book and travel, in stillness, to far-off places and witness incidents in the imaginary lives of others. Reading is not so easily escapist, nor should we wish it to be, and I can't in fact tell you about the books without telling you about the cancer. The story we read in a novel meets, in our minds, the experiences of our own lives, and something substantial forms. The stories converse with one another, and with ourselves; far from being an escape from life, they help us to live it more deeply. As do, at times, the stories that come to us in the course of the day – through the internet, the newspaper, the evening bulletin, the voices of people we love – which can be just as sustaining as those we read in books.

I was still trying to think through my diagnosis when a friend was called to her doctor's surgery to hear the results of her own cancer tests. I asked which of her daughters she would take with her, knowing from experience how bad it could be to wait, afraid.

'None,' she said. 'I'm going on my own. I've got a book.'

I wish I'd asked what she was reading. Charles Dickens? She was a big fan of Dickens. *Bleak House*? Now that's something to occupy the most nervous hands.

I first learned about diseases of the breast more than ten years ago, in Palo Alto. I was writing a novel about Edgar Allan Poe at the time, and was working my way through Stanford University's collection of Poe material. I slept in a hotel room that fitted me like a nutshell. At night I sat cross-legged on the bed with my books in front of me. Down in the lobby, there was excellent coffee, back issues of *The New Yorker*, and, near the foot of an old lift made of brass and wood and glass reinforced with chicken wire, a piano.

Someone was always playing the piano, and from time to time the desk clerk would dart across the great expanse of shabby flooring to explain that this was not allowed. It made no difference; insomniac pianists disobeyed him, and Chopin drifted up the lift-well to my room.

By day I walked to the university, where I had another room, on the first floor of a research institute. It had been a house once, the elegant clapboard retirement home of the first president of the university, who lived on the campus into old age. I've always loved wooden houses, the way they take in wind and sound. Footfalls are different in a wooden house. My university room had plenty of shelving and a small desk that a child, perhaps a grandchild of the president, might once have used. Here, in the daytime, I did my work on Poe.

Edgar Allan Poe wrote about men who cannot steady their minds; about ailing women, frail in life yet active, killingly capable, after they die. Sometimes they don't have to lift a finger, these dead women. Their men mourn so terribly, are fearfully alone, deranged, busy with self-destruction. There is no recovery; Poe's characters do not, in the cruel and shallow phrasing of our own time, move on and form new relationships. Grief is not like that.

These days we've turned our faces to the wall in the matter of death and loss. We're just not looking. In the nineteenth century people couldn't look away. One of Poe's literary rivals, Rufus Griswold, remained with his wife's corpse for thirty hours. He's quoted as saying: 'I kiss her cold lips, but their fervour is gone.' I'm not sure what he expected. Something more than simple extinction? We all expect more than that.

At Stanford I was reading everything I could about death in the nineteenth century, but I lived in a twentieth-century haven of comfort and good company. The shelves in my room were full of books written by the women at the research institute, and one of them was Marilyn Yalom's *A History of the Breast*.

What stayed in my mind over the following years was one of her epigraphs, by the Spanish writer Ramón Gómez de la Serna: 'When poets speak of death, they call it the place "without breasts".' In Yalom's book I read about nursing mothers, about pornographers, about political displays of the breast by revolutionaries and liberationists. I saw the breasts of the Virgin as the painter Jean Fouquet imagined them: high and spherical with small blank nipples. I read about breast cancer with detached concern. It was terrible, but remote. Nobody I knew had ever had it. It didn't happen to women like me, or so I thought, fit women with no family history of cancer. Women who were disciplined about food and exercise.

Like the character Lauren Hartke in Don DeLillo's novel *The Body Artist*, I 'worked my body hard', in the swimming pool and on the walking track. Lauren is 'the dictator' of her body, and I too had confidence in the health and submission of my physical self. It did what it was told.

When I read about those women with breast cancer I thought, Poor souls. It's a phrase my grandmother used. She never spoke of happy souls. The soul was always pitiful, it seemed, and when a person was in difficulty you looked to the suffering of their spirit.

Back in Australia I tucked a copy of *A History of the Breast* on my shelf and it slept there until I suddenly, badly, needed it.

Just before I was told I had cancer I saw a strange exhibition. A German artist, Wolfgang Laib, was showing his work at the gallery in my university. For me, his most impressive pieces were squares of softly luminous yellow pollen, sieved into carpet-shaped sections on the floor. I looked down at this simple and absorbing colour. It was deeply soothing art, without perspective, without the need for the eye to travel, for the mind to entirely understand. There were no distractions, just pure colour. Laib was also showing sculptures made of stone and beeswax which had the slight perfume of late-night conversations when the candles burn low.

Wolfgang Laib was once a doctor and apparently feels that he has never stopped being a doctor. I don't know exactly what his art might remedy. Human disproportion and loneliness, perhaps. The big illnesses, bigger than cancers and worn-out hearts.

Cancer is said to give its sufferers a sense of proportion, but for me everything just went horribly flat. I felt perpetually lightly stunned. It was calming, in a way. In Tolstoy's *Anna Karenina* Levin thinks that 'there's less charm in life, when one thinks about death, but there's more peace'. It would be a pleasure, this freedom from everyday emotion, if only the ordinary were not replaced by solitary, constant fear. But although I felt alone I had plenty of company. A GP once told me that in her practice cancer was almost as common as the flu.

'It's a big tumour,' my own GP said. 'And you'll need all the support you can get.' That's when it came, the simultaneous sense of falling and of being crushed. I was thinking about my son. He was fourteen then, and I had sole responsibility for his day-to-day care. For his meals, laundry and homework, for getting him to school and tennis lessons. In earlier years I had made up answers to questions about the mechanics of jet propulsion, the habits of komodo dragons and God. I was the safety officer in the family, the person who dealt with difficulties and anxiety. And now I was suddenly weak with fear. I was not going to be able to fix this. We were not safe at all.

There's no provision for the protection of children in a cancer diagnosis, but I knew, urgently, that I couldn't leave him. My son. He was my field of pollen, and the sense of him stayed in my mind like a colour after my eyes were closed. I asked the doctor if I would live.

'Yes,' he said. 'I believe so.' He was entirely confident, although really he couldn't know. He wrote me a script for Valium, for the fearful times when I wasn't sitting in his surgery in the full light of his confidence. He had swum the English Channel in a relay; there were photos of it in the waiting room. He knew what he was doing.

I drove home from the surgery that morning and I couldn't sit and I couldn't stand still. All the small things I once enjoyed had suddenly lost meaning and power. What was the point of my photographs, my books, my precious things? If I didn't survive this, my son would look at them alone. Was there any point at all in a porcelain Chinese pillow shaped like a cat, bought in an antique shop in Charlottesville, Virginia? Someone long dead had dreamed on it. Every trace of their thought, their breath and memory had disappeared. Only the human mattered, and the human was so quickly gone.

I was demolished, stupid with grief and fear. I paced swiftly, arms folded, from one window to another.

Somewhere I had read or heard that a particular French executioner had a trick to help the condemned take up their position on the scaffold. As he led them forward he told them to mind the step, so that they looked at their feet and not up at the blade of the guillotine. The small fear of tripping preoccupied them briefly and they were able to move sensibly to their deaths. For a time I was like a prisoner who had looked up instead of down, a prisoner who had glimpsed the blade. I was terrified. Then I calmed enough to phone my father in the east. His voice was steady, questioning me, thinking ahead to the next step: telling my mother.

Of course the news destroyed them temporarily. The eldest of my two brothers later told me they looked as if they had been shot. I felt deeply guilty for causing them such pain. I felt ashamed.

And then I started thinking about the steps I must take, all those light, sure-footed steps away from death toward the medical world. Toward a sense of purpose, even hope.

Our grandparents or great-grandparents usually had a bookshelf with an encyclopaedia, novels, poetry and a medical guide, perhaps *Ladies' Handbook of Home Treatment*, which my grandmother had owned since girlhood. It instructed her on how to treat ailments and broken bones, how to fumigate a room following a death from tuberculosis, how to wrap and bake a piece of cloth for use as sterile dressings after childbirth.

She kept this book to hand into the television age, well into the age of major public hospitals equipped for the most adventurous surgery and post-operative care. It sat on her shelf with Dickens and Walter Scott, and just before she died she copied out Tennyson's poem, 'Crossing the Bar'. My mother has the handwritten page: 'Sunset and evening star,/And one clear call for me!/And may there be no moaning of the bar,/When I put out to sea . . .' The bookshelf of that era was restorative, and it was no accident that medicine and literature leaned against one another, offering direction.

I was very lucky in my education. When I was nineteen I read Samuel Beckett with my tutor, who was old, Buddhist, kind. His room smelled of paper, it smelled of stone and autumn. For three hours each week we read aloud to one another, taking a turn when the voice of the other fell silent, murmuring the work like music. We were not reading in pursuit of a plot, we were listening. We read from Beckett's trilogy, *Molloy*, *Malone Dies* and *The Unnamable*.

Beckett was Irish, although he lived in France for much of his life and wrote his greatest work in French, including the trilogy, which was then translated back into Irish-inflected English. The Ireland in his fiction is stony and ungiving. His characters too are desperate, ancient, filthy, solitary, forceful men, but they're described with great comic vigour. They are captivating, these characters, a pleasure for the reader not because they're appealing in themselves, but because the writing makes them so. Beckett's work can be difficult to read, since it's as involved with the problems of storytelling as with telling a story, but the trilogy is also funny and hypnotic. The vagrants and lost men who are his protagonists in these three novels have nothing with which to entertain themselves, and us, but a brilliant display of words.

When you read aloud from the trilogy, in the right room, in the right light, it's possible to slip into a calm state that has nothing to do with resignation. There is a particular music in his sentences, and this can shift the reader's mood into something like entrancement. In the trilogy he makes a joke of true love, but he doesn't reduce it to rubble. And in *Malone Dies* he shows us that there can be something apart from helplessness and despair in waiting for the end of a life, the end of a story.

When Beckett was very old, too frail to live independently, he took a few possessions to his room in a nursing home. One of them was a copy of Dante's *The Divine Comedy* that he had owned for more than sixty years. It was perhaps the book of his life. *Malone Dies* became one of the books of my life. I never tire of reading it; it steadies me, as Dante may have steadied Beckett, as Tennyson's sunset and evening star steadied my grandmother.

You set sail in starlight. You leave the harbour for the ocean. Guided by a strange pilot, you pass into the night. This is death, as Tennyson imagines it, and when I think about that time in my life, that time of cancer surgery, I also think of the sea, which brings us the rhythm of the waves, the weightless pleasure of flotation, but also, if we're unlucky, engulfment and death.

There's a kind of fish that sleeps in a bubble, an envelope of shiny material that flows from its mouth like soft wet glass and surrounds it, to protect it from minor predators. Outside lie the terrors of the reef. Inside, the fish sleeps alone and open-eyed. Perhaps it isn't sleeping. Perhaps it lies in an unimaginable fish-trance. The fish may be a little blinded by its glossy envelope.

If a reef shark finds this envelope it bites deeply into the fish, flinging its head from side to side so that the churn of water and the snapping motion help tear the fish apart.

I saw all this on television, and despite the matter-of-fact tone of the narrator, I was a little shocked. I felt a connection with the fish in its trance, looking out at a distorted world. The things that issue from our mouths are so ineffectual in the face of destruction.

I have been interested for so many years in human wreckage. I have observed it as a writer. I have tried not to make my writing shiny or self-protective, but the act of writing creates a sweet enclosure for the ego. It's difficult, yes, solitary, but so very sweet. I didn't ever imagine that the reef shark would come for me. When it did I reached for my old defences: solitude, the light state of the writer's trance. Holding that sense of trance in waiting rooms. Perhaps at some level I still thought I was invulnerable, looking out through a clear barrier into the blackness of the reef, where the wreckage of strangers' bodies lay.

I'd been in hospital once before my cancer surgery, to have a baby. I knew from that experience how a body can recover from a great distorting transformation, and when I gathered my thoughts I decided to think of the cancer as a difficult pregnancy. At the end of it would be a new human life: my own.

My real pregnancy happened in 1990, during the First Gulf War. Suddenly I was in the zone of killing and creating, war and motherhood. Just before the conflict broke out I went to a peace service at a cathedral in the city. I was given a candle with a cardboard collar that someone had carefully fashioned to protect my fingers from hot wax. There were Quakers, Buddhists, Anglicans, a row of elderly Irish nuns. Everyone in the congregation had a candle with a cardboard ledge, everyone was hopeful, but our hopes came to nothing; the war began.

I'm a youngest child, without sisters; I didn't know a lot about pregnancy and childbirth. I asked my mother what it was like to have a baby. 'All the points of the compass swivel,' she told me. She meant that I'd have to reorient myself or I'd be lost, and she was right. When I asked my hairdresser what to expect she said, 'Imagine cutting off your own leg.'

After my baby was born, he began to gasp and cry out and fling his hands up, arms wide in a gesture of surrender – a startled reflex that brought to mind the victim facing the firing squad in Goya's *The Shootings of May Third.* That same frozen astonishment. My son's face was thick-featured from all the fluid he'd been swimming in. He would never have this underwater face again. By the time we were settled in a big public ward, he looked much like all the other babies in their wire baskets beside their mothers' beds. He deteriorated over the next few days; he was yellow, listless, baggy-skinned. He failed to thrive.

The ward was full. One of the women, a refugee who'd had a long labour and whose baby was unsettled, spent a lot of time looking out the window. Her baby cried and cried, and when this mother was offered painkillers for herself, a binder for her breasts, she refused. 'Oh, doesn't matter,' she said. 'One or two days sore.'

My baby and I didn't thrive until we were allowed home and I was tucked into my high wooden bed with him in the curve of my arm, his father bringing me fish and salad. The marriage didn't last, but it was good for a very long time. As I drifted off to sleep my husband played the piano in a distant room. In the night the baby and I turned about each other like the planets.

In the daytime I was listening to a radio reading of Nabokov's *Invitation to a Beheading*, a novel that suited the larger anxieties of the time. Military jets were flying through European skies on their way to Iraq. My nights with a sleepy baby seemed so vast and orderly, but that was the illusion of maternal self-absorption; the forces in the wider world seemed to be given over to destruction. And so it seemed important to keep listening to Nabokov's novel.

Invitation to a Beheading domesticates state-sanctioned killing and portrays the sense of righteous purpose that makes it possible. A man, Cincinnatus, has been condemned for a crime that isn't specified. As he waits for the day of his execution people appear in his cell, exaggerating their roles: his faithless wife brings her lover, her family and even furniture with her when she visits; his mother makes small talk and urges him to eat the sweets she's brought; the executioner himself turns up, sensible and overfriendly.

Contrasting with all this drama is the prisoner's simple understanding of what death entails. Cincinnatus has the terrible human regret that we all feel in the face of our own extinction. Death is such a waste of an intricate human body. ' "I have been fashioned so painstakingly," thought Cincinnatus as he wept in the darkness. "The curvature of my spine has been calculated so well, so mysteriously. I feel, tightly rolled up in my calves, so many miles that I could yet run in my lifetime. My head is so comfortable . . ." '

Leaving this body will be like climbing out of bed in winter. ' "But now I don't want to die! My soul has burrowed under the pillow. Oh, I don't want to! It will be cold getting out of my warm body. I don't want to . . . wait a while . . . let me doze some more." ' It's a childish and deeply understandable plea.

In the end the prisoner and the executioner, the latter with his axe and his assistant, ride to the scaffold together. The executioner deals with Cincinnatus with firm, parental authority. What is most chilling is the soothing tone he uses to correct him, as he tries to protect the back of his neck with his hands. The French executioner who told his victims to mind the step so they wouldn't be paralysed by the sight of the guillotine above was mimicking parental concern in much the same way.

When women with an older style of mothering told me that my baby was spoiled, that babies should be trained from the moment they're born, I heard the faint echo of the voice of grim limitation, the voice of power organising a helpless person for their own convenience, and with the help of Nabokov, an unlikely adviser on childcare, I resisted. His Cincinnatus, 'fashioned so painstakingly', captures the sense of reverent wonder about the human body that loving parents feel on examining their babies. I didn't believe that my baby's body was the only thing to have been painstakingly fashioned – I had confidence that his demands were as necessary to him as his respiration, his circulatory system, and all his other biological processes, and I felt no need to train what had been so intricately put together and delivered to me.

As my son grew older I taught him the ABC. I read him stories, we made words with a plastic alphabet, and we had a chart with letters and pictures, beginning with an apple, a bird, a clown. In the book *Norah's Ark* a woman saves her animals from a flood by upturning their barn and building a shelter in the watertight roof. She sits on her tractor with one fist raised, her animals lifted above the dark water. Norah and the animals play I Spy to pass the time. W is for water. My son and I spelled out 'ark' and 'water' with our plastic lettering. We read about Norah and as we spelled out letters the flood was defeated, the animals were saved. How soothing it is to read a story a syllable at a time. How different from the coercive voice of the executioner, persuading the prisoner to position himself for death.

I was once seated next to a young heart surgeon at a wedding reception and of course I asked him how it felt to cut into the human heart.

'Just like any meat,' he replied, as I expected. Then, with the skill of a poet, or a flirt, he added, 'Just like any meat, but softer.'

And I remembered that my mother, when I was fifteen and miserable, sent me not to a psychiatrist but to a heart surgeon, who listened and spoke to me kindly, understanding, in all ways, the florid tenderness of the adolescent heart.

I have a friend who abandoned surgery and became a GP after a bitter quarrel with a more senior doctor. He tells me that his work in general practice involves his patients' stories as well as their bodies. A person arrives in his rooms with a story that they have had time – often considerable time – to develop, and he must quickly and correctly grasp its often hidden import and match it to the story that his profession provides for the purpose. Some patients are duplicitous, angling for drugs or personal attachment.

In my own GP's waiting room I see girls in school uniform, glossy pregnant women, and young men with teeth that have been destroyed by amphetamines. I think about my doctor sitting behind his broad desk, nimbly interpreting stories I can only guess at. The imagination flourishes in the everyday practice of medicine as well as in fiction, and sometimes in the latter it's not only the patients who present themselves inventively, calculatingly.

In *Bleak House*, Dickens portrays several doctors whose attitudes to their work could not be less alike. Skimpole is selfish and indolent and fearful of infection; he's also a sponger (his character is based on the impoverished poet Leigh Hunt). Young Richard Carstone begins medical training but he throws it in, it's 'uphill work'. The surgeon Alan Woodcourt, by contrast, is close to poverty, working out in the slums, in the squalid rooms of his patients. Finally he is forced by his straitened circumstances to put to sea as a ship's doctor.

This means he must farewell Esther, the narrator of *Bleak House*, who is so modest in her tones, so insistent on her own plainness, so eloquent about the loveliness of her friend Ada, that we might be surprised to discover she is the illegitimate daughter of a great society beauty and therefore quite possibly attractive herself. While Woodcourt is out of the country Esther falls ill. She survives, but her face is scarred. When they meet again, almost by accident, she misreads Woodcourt. She thinks he pities her. He does, but he's also in love with her.

She tells us with sweet formality, 'I felt as if he had greater commiseration for me than I had ever had for myself.' In the novel we see Woodcourt less as a lover than a doctor, and Esther might be speaking for all the desolate people he tends. His compassion is at the heart of his medical work. He cares more about his patients than they care about themselves. It must be uphill work indeed.

One of my anaesthetists was a smoker. As I lay on various operating tables, my arm outstretched while he tried for a difficult vein, feeling afraid and repeating to myself the words of the refugee in the maternity ward – 'It doesn't matter, one or two days sore' – I used to imagine him in the evenings, in some courtyard, rolling himself a cigarette. The first cigarette of the night: delicious.

I know this because I smoked a lot as a student in Canberra, where the cold winters seemed to encourage it. I stopped when I came to live in Western Australia. My anaesthetist understood what he risked; he looked down on surgically opened chests and cancerous lungs. He too could one day be lying on a narrow bench, afraid, inventing stories to make it easier for another human being to pierce his flesh. I would think about this for the few seconds before his drugs took me under.

But I wasn't responsible for his health. I'm not a doctor, I don't deal directly with such human concerns daily, hourly, for a living.

I'm writing about good doctors because I had good doctors. I know that some are careless, or harsh, or simply tired – the spirit of Dickens' character Skimpole isn't confined to the pages of an old book. But my doctors were good, and I don't believe their goodness was exceptional.

It all began, this whole medical adventure, with the expression on a stranger's face. I was lying on a bed next to an ultrasound machine while the technician slid her implement over the gel on my skin. She was watching the monitor and I was watching her. This technician, and the man who later performed the biopsy with his hollow needles, were bad actors. Their faces gave too much away.

Further up the medical hierarchy, you find a different level of acting skill. Later, when my oncologist pressed her fingers into my throat, feeling for irregular lymph nodes, I asked, 'How do I know if you've found something bad?'

She had a firm, painless touch. 'If I find something bad my smile might fade,' she said. 'Or it might not.'

At the point when I was lying on the bed for an ultrasound, I didn't know I was going to need an oncologist. I knew I was tired all the time, that I had a long ribbon of pain down one side of my throat. Something was wrong with me, I just wasn't sure what. I was working hard at the university and I was finishing a book, I had plenty of reasons to be tired. Writing, when it's going well, can drive away all that is outside the page, outside the small territory of the author's obsession. But my writing wasn't going well. My novel was about the First World War, and I was often too tired to try to revive the past.

I'd attempted to cure myself with good food, sunshine, a short holiday on Rottnest Island where you can swim, cycle on paths through sand dunes and salt plains, or go to the museum displaying the history of the island. I went with the man I was seeing at the time. Our hotel room overlooked a pink lake; it was late summer, warm. I opened the shutters and switched on the overhead fan, made a meal of tea and melon. Quokkas came looking for treats. Other guests fed them chocolate from the minibar – they weren't impressed by healthy fruit. In the sea, stingrays flew slowly through the deeper water and the current pulled all the anchored boats into perfect lines. Children in brightly coloured T-shirts stamped on the wet sand, each step displacing the water and leaving a brief dry footprint. I tried to ignore the fact that I was feeling strange, exhausted.

Some months later, I finally saw my GP. I showed him an odd dimple on my skin and he sent me for preliminary investigations to rule out breast cancer. Except they didn't rule it out. I saw the face of the woman who was watching the ultrasound screen and I knew in an instant.

There followed the vertigo-inducing appointment with my GP, then another with the surgeon who was to remove the tumour, quick conversations on the telephone to organise leave from work, hours of immobility as I sat numbly, and periods of rushing through household tasks to make up for the time I'd lost sitting still. Nine days of fear – until I found myself hesitating before an unzipped carry-bag in my upstairs room, wondering which book to take to hospital. The man I was involved with was visiting his family in America at this stage, and by the time he returned, everything between us had changed. It was over.

I was proud of my independence, proud of my family of two. Mother and child: the smallest possible family. It worked well, as long as the grown-up member had health and energy, but now we were confronting changes that would require great mental and financial steadying. We were lucky we weren't alone: we were isolated, here in Western Australia, but we sprang from a big steady family in the east, people of quick initiative, who were suddenly facing the possible death of a daughter and sister.

I have an old book on my shelves, *The Tosa Diary*. It was written more than a thousand years ago, in Japanese, and published in English translation in 1912. So very old, so far from lost. It's a kind of travel book, written by Ki No Tsurayuki, a provincial governor. He uses the language of women, which was the voice of the vernacular, the non-literary. He's describing a sea journey to Kyoto at the end of his period of service, and something rises from the page as sharply as the smell of salt and seaweed and the washed bones of seabirds. The language is so ancient that the translation cannot come close to exactness; we must find him with our senses.

The Tosa Diary came into my hands when I was staying with a friend in Sydney, sleeping on a couch in her study. I wake early and she likes to sleep through the morning, so I had hours to fill before the day began. The diary was shelved at the same height as my pillow. The spine caught my eye and I reached for it and started to read as dawn broke and the sky outside turned rose and white and blue.

Later, when I began to take more notice of Japanese literature and art, I came across the dawn sky in the works of the famous nineteenth-century artist Hiroshige. His woodblock prints frequently show a sky white at the horizon with dawn mist, blotted above with an intense and darkening blue. For me Japanese art, like no other visual art, is associated with natural transitions, particularly sunrise, when the sky changes with swift dramatic ease. There is a lesson in this. As you watch the light being released into darkness you understand that change can be great and ordinary all at once. Dawn is a time of release, and also, for me, a time to read and think, before the active day.

Reading, too, is a release, sometimes flooded with illumination.

There's a place, of course, for systematic reading, for gathering information on a specific subject, but Japanese books always seemed to come to me fortuitously, gifts of chance or accident, as a result of loitering in bookshops, libraries, before the shelves of friends. In a famous fourteenth-century Japanese text called *Essays in Idleness*, the writer, a Buddhist priest, tells us: 'The pleasantest of all diversions is to sit alone under the lamp, a book spread out before you, and to make friends with people of a distant past you have never known.'

Drawing close to distant characters, inviting them to join our contemporary stories of illness and travel and children, of love and anxiety, confirms the work of our lives, which is surely to look beyond ourselves, for companionship, or else to brace against those people and situations better considered at a distance. For not every character we meet in books is friendly, and some stories are filled with darkness.

My friend gave me *The Tosa Diary* as I stood on the landing outside her apartment, an overnight bag at my feet, a ride to the airport and a long flight ahead of me. This book was the beginning of my wanderings in the literature of Japan. The storyteller in it is an almost compulsive poet, but the exchange of formal verse seems to be part of the courtesies of the time and place. He writes of the reflection of the moon on water, and the strange likeness of sea foam to snow, or spring flowers, although we know that the boat is on the open sea, pursued by pirates.

This is no ship's log, it has the poise and simplicity of art. The diarist writes poetry not only out of good manners or in response to the natural world, but because the story is flooded with sadness, and poetry suits the mood. A child has died, and must be left behind. In one poem she is compared to a pearl. Ki No Tsurayuki adds a few lines after the poem: 'Thus he spoke in memory of his little daughter, for a parent is apt to become very childish. Some may object that she was not like a pearl; be that as it may, the child is dead, and it is no empty compliment to say she had a beautiful face.'

The journal finishes with a dismissive comment that we can't possibly agree with, and surely its writer doesn't want us to: 'His sorrows, which he can never forget, are more than he can ever express. Well, well, – this must be torn up at once.' The traveller must put grief aside, or, if that is beyond him, and it clearly is, the diary itself must be destroyed.

I see, in *The Tosa Diary*, the space of vital regret where a daughter should be.

We all slip away from home, we all voyage with some adult purpose, and we all, somehow, fail to leave. We return to the distant members of our family in thoughts and dreams, which are everyone's internal, silent poetry, and never more often or more impatiently than in illness or near death.

When I read *The Tosa Diary* I thought of my father, of what he did when I was small to keep his family afloat. He worked on the land that had been owned by his own father, and when I was little I rode on his shoulders, high above the powdery dust on the track between the farmhouse and the main road, above his pastures, cornfields and black cattle. We lived in the house my grandfather had built above a riverbank.

The novelist E.M. Forster writes: 'a wonderful physical tie binds the parents to the children; and – by some sad strange irony – it does not bind us children to our parents'. He imagines the possibilities 'if we could answer their love not with gratitude but with equal love'. The entrancement, the concern, the intuition of a parent can't be neatly returned. But I don't think it's lost.

My father taught me that staring directly at an object in the dark can make it seem to blur, even to move a little, frighteningly. He said that the best way to see anything in the dark is to relax, and to fix your gaze on a point next to the frightening thing. It works: a shape of sick horror becomes clothes thrown over the back of a chair. My father repeated this advice throughout my childhood, and he tucked me into bed with hands which will always be broader than mine, and which are marked, on the palms, with a few deep lines in clear directions, not like the confusion of fine, splitting lines on my own.

It seems to me that for Forster, we humans stand in a column, loving the child in front of us, who will grow with their back to us and will in time love the child in front of them, who turns their back to love their own, and so on. But is he right? Am I taking the time to write this, I ask myself, with my back to my father?

In Isaiah the Lord says, 'I have made you and I will bear the burden, I will carry you and bring you to safety.' It's a statement of patriarchal confidence, so confident we might almost expect some ironic reversal, some dropping of the baby. But cynical expectations can be wrong; my own father carried us to safety during a flood, when the house was submerged and the cattle were swept away in the water.

I have a memory of silver light on the ripples of a fast black current. I sit on the floor of a boat with my father at the oars, my brothers and mother on benches just above me. I can see out across the dark water, over the rim of the boat. The crowns of trees are breaking through the surface, snagging drowned cattle and corrugated iron. Perhaps there is a bright moon, perhaps my mother is shining a powerful torch out over the water. We skim and pause, and skim again.

The doors of the house on the riverbank have been left open, my mother's piano raised out of reach of the water which will soon pour down the hallway and through the rooms. The flood is at the very lip of the kitchen door when I step into the boat and settle, for stability, on the bottom.

Earlier that night, the river had risen so quickly that our boat, tethered to a willow tree that was rapidly being engulfed, was almost submerged. My father dived from what was left of the bank and followed the rope down to the trunk of the tree. I think of him, alone and blind in the pull of the black water, lungs bursting, dragging himself further down, fist over fist along a rope which must be untied before we can be saved.

All my life I've dreamed of currents closing behind me as I walk along a sandbar, of mirrors collapsing into torrents of water. I'm in a house that holds firm in the tunnel of a wave. I'm holding my child up to admire his reflection when the mirror splits in a hiss of spray and cracks under the pressure of interior water.

In my memory my father is diving for the boat and I'm waiting with the others on my mother's polished kitchen floor, practising looking next to things in the darkened rooms, beyond the candlelight. We're waiting for the sound of the dipping oars, for my father to prevail against the black current and steady the boat at the kitchen door and reach for us, one by one. Once he's settled us in the boat, he rows calmly across the bright surface of the water and we need not concern ourselves with whatever lies beneath.

I don't want to leave him, bereaved like the father in *The Tosa Diary*.

And then there's my mother. As I stared at my unzipped bag, wondering which book to take to hospital, my mother was on an aeroplane. Nobody, she believes, should wake from an anaesthetic alone.

When we discussed the cancer surgery I said, 'At least it's me. At least it isn't my child.'

There was a slight hesitation before she said, 'But you are *my* child.'

Imagine an empty hospital bed in a dark room. A black and white television at the foot of the bed casts light on the coverlet. Stars are projected in a soft blur across the walls. A face appears on one of the walls, a woman's. Her features, too, are soft and indistinct. You watch the stars, the face and the hospital bed in this enchanted room, listening to a rushing wind.

I stood in such a space in 2009. It was an installation called 'In the Shadow of Stars', part of an exhibition by the Australian artist Ken Unsworth, in memory of his wife, the pianist Elisabeth, who'd died the previous year. The installation used Elisabeth's hospital bed, a relic of her illness, and was set up in a disused turbine room on Cockatoo Island, in Sydney Harbour. The ferry that took me there passed under the bridge, its great arc nubbled with the bodies of healthy climbers. On the island, oysters sat at the waterline; dark gold kelp like shredded tobacco moved slowly below the surface.

The stillness of Elisabeth's bedside, re-created in her husband's art, was quite a change from the harbour. But it wasn't a sombre place, it was loving. The pale moving lights of the projected galaxies shone above the metal tubing of the bed. I grew very familiar with hospital beds between 2005 and 2008, each one a little raft between the islands of the admission desk and the operating theatre; a small platform for waiting, at times in pain, at times in a state of sadness, for the momentary surge of hope.

The hospital where I had cancer surgery was nothing like the basic public ward where I had my baby. I felt as if I'd come to a European hotel. There was a crowd, like a tour group, in front of the admission desk. Small suitcases. Tired murmurings.

I was taken to a room with a narrow bed, a bed the width of a gutter, where a technician injected a dye that would show which lymph nodes the blood from the cancer site entered. These nodes would then be removed during surgery and examined by a pathologist. If they contained cancer cells, my chances of survival would diminish.

The hospital was built on a sliver of land between an escarpment and a road. As images of my veins were being taken I looked out at a wall of rock and eucalypts, the familiar, undramatic shadings of the Australian bush and a view of the sky, for which I was so thankful. It was a day when other people drove to work, flicked through emails, dealt with real and electronic in-trays. Did things. Got about. I was shown to my ward, helpless, meditative, obedient, and soon I would be unconscious. I was going to have to get used to this new condition.

As I rolled on the pressure stockings that would prevent my body developing thrombosis during the long period of inactivity under anaesthetic, I thought of the white legs of a Japanese doll, stiff and still. The hospital gown, tied with loose pragmatic bows, was designed for swift removal but I would be unaware of this. I would be completely unaware.

After the surgery someone leaned close to my face and whispered that I was safe, it was over, and no cancerous cells had been found in my lymph nodes. And then she said it again, more loudly, for my mother to hear.

The surgeon was less cheerful. Cancer, he told us, can slip through the blood undetected. He thought it would be wise to have chemotherapy and radiotherapy.

It was nine days since my GP had told me I had cancer. In a month and a half I would begin chemotherapy. Six treatments, with three-week recovery periods between each one. And following that, daily radiation.

As I recovered from surgery I watched the bubbles in the thin tube of saline that was taped above the vein in my arm. Tiny, glassy circles of air. I was looking, as my father had instructed me, to one side in the dark. For a time I couldn't seem to pull my eyes into alignment, I couldn't read. But I could listen to my iPod. My son had chosen the music. My heart seemed to strengthen, to feed on the rhythm of a bass line.

The day after the operation, the Anglican priest who had baptised my son fourteen years before came to sit on the edge of my bed. He took my hands in his. I closed my eyes and he quoted a line from a poem by David Campbell: 'Praise life while you walk and wake – it is only lent.' I misunderstood. I thought he was talking about Lent, the period of fasting and austerity in the liturgical calendar. I was in a lean time, I told myself. A time before some season of celebration.

When he left I did a little hospital housekeeping. Folded my things. Emptied vases and culled wilted flowers. I moved carefully, because I had to carry and settle the vacuum bottle that conveyed fluid from the surgery site. The bottle was like a dull baby. Like a cold, unhappy pet. It needed looking after. My day was full of domestic responsibilities.

Then at last I was dressed, released, or at least free of the hospital, a seatbelt across my painful chest, the view from a road I had driven along for years now looking strange, as if the far bank of the Swan River were suddenly more distant, as if whole trees had been planted, or taken away, while I was gone.

And what, finally, had I taken with me to read? Beckett, of course. And I took the page proofs of my novel to the hospital.

I corrected it on the bed table, manoeuvring it over the covers, using the hand that wasn't complicated with tape and plastic tubing. Seeing the final design of a book you've written can be so satisfying; in a distant city, strangers had taken care in the way they set my words down on the page. 'Live and invent,' writes Malone in *Malone Dies*, although he does wonder if he's chosen the right words. As I worked I thought, too, of a comment Saul Bellow makes in his novel *Ravelstein*: 'I am a great believer in the power of unfinished work to keep you alive.' Write, my books were telling me. Live.

An immense and shaggy man, partially paralysed, lies alone in a bed in a single room with a closed door and a sealed window. This is Malone, of *Malone Dies*. He has a view of rooftops and the sky; he can see a pair of lovers who forgot to draw their blind. Strange hands leave him food and lift away his pot of waste, and then this ceases. He never sees a face. He has a pencil and a notebook and he tells himself stories that he doesn't believe, while he waits to die.

In these stories a French peasant enslaves and butchers his animals and his family. A couple bicker about a pen. Malone is a writer at work, he continuously doubles back on his characters, commenting, revising, pushing them forward and shrugging them off. We can hear his pencil sliding across the page because he tells us exactly how it feels to write. From time to time he describes his few possessions; he clings, in particular, to a stick.

What is it that so appeals to me about a single room? A bedroom with a writing desk, a hotel room, or the space below deck on a well-fitted boat, even a hospital room. They're places of privacy and sufficiency, where everything you need is close at hand. In Florence, years ago, I had a room with shuttered windows which opened above a market near the Medici Chapel. Someone had given me lilacs at the railway station. At certain times of the day the green of the shutters exactly matched the colour of their leaves. It was a place to read and think after a long flight and a journey by train. One of the perfect single rooms.

When I was a child my grandmother bought me painted marzipan fruit in a nest of straw from Naples. I found the same kind of sweet more than twenty years later in Florence, and in that perfect room I broke apart a marzipan peach, sitting cross-legged on my narrow bed, wrapped in the smell of almond and sugar, solitary yet safe as an animal in the Ark.

There's no lilac in Malone's room. His door is unlocked. Someone terrible visits him, watches him for a time, attacks him, leaves, comes back, watches again and finally disappears. Malone keeps making up stories.

His last is a story about Macmann, a vagrant in an asylum, horribly in love with his ancient dying nurse, Moll, who encourages his passion and tries to fetch oysters for aphrodisiac feasts.

She wears crucifix earrings, and her sole tooth is carved into the shape of a cross. The earrings, she explains, are the thieves who were crucified with Jesus; the tooth is the Redeemer, imprisoned in her mouth. She's not an obvious romantic heroine.

Macmann's love poetry might just be the worst in the language. He loses Moll. But we recognise Macmann: he is Malone in love, Malone in a single room with what passes for food and passion, mobile enough to wander in a shabby garden, *compos* enough to know where exactly he is, and possibly why. Together their names include the words *man* and *alone*. They spell out Malone's sad situation.

After Moll's death she is replaced by a much more unpleasant nurse, Lemuel, who sleeps and eats on the bare boards of his own empty room, steals the solids in the lunatics' soup, beats himself with a hammer, and hands Macmann over to even more brutal staff for punishment. There's no talk of love, no poetry.

At the end of the story, Macmann and his fellow inmates are loaded into a boat for a picnic organised by a charitable aristocrat. A journey over water, in poetry and mythology, signifies a journey into death. There is no picnic. Lemuel uses a hatchet to slaughter the lunatics, the aristocrat and the boatmen.

Lemuel, the executioner, governs the bewildered Macmann, imprisons him, releases him, and destroys him without any reason, except that the story must be resolved, and quickly, as Malone the writer is at the point of death.

Why take a deathbed novel into cancer surgery? Why steer straight into the dark?

Alberto Manguel, in *A History of Reading*, points out the appeal of reading something as far from your own surroundings as possible. 'For [the writer] Colette, *Les Misérables*, with its streets and forests, flights down dark sewers and across battling barricades, was the perfect book for the quiet of the bedroom.' There's something to be said for a book that contrasts with the reader's own experience, but I don't think this notion is more than a guiding principle.

For me, *Malone Dies* was the right book for the hospital bed because it is drenched in regret. Malone has almost no possessions, no parents to farewell, no children, no real home. No personal distractions. Just sorrow at the loss of the final pure things: thought and memory and story. This is what you lose when you lose your life, and the loss is incalculable. Malone writes of the 'soul denied in vain, vigilant, anxious, turning in its cage as in a lantern, in the night without haven or craft or matter or understanding'. Poor soul, as my grandmother would say, helpless, trapped, unsupported. Malone's lament is a moment of sympathy, and perhaps belief.

Some degree of trust and faith are required just to make our way in the day-to-day world, but I like to read books that touch on a stronger belief, that show us ways other people deal with the problem of meaning. Don DeLillo writes about religious faith in his novel *Falling Man*, where one character finds God in stained-glass windows and the music of Bach. Beckett doesn't seem to have had religious beliefs, but biblical stories and great poems of faith can still speak powerfully to the non-believer. Folded into *Malone Dies,* that most bleak of deathbed novels, is Dante's *The Divine Comedy*, a most deeply imagined work of love and faith. We don't have to accept the idea of a Christian heaven in order to believe that Dante's afterlife can give beauty and direction to our existence.

In Florence, Dante's birthplace, I found myself before a fresco depicting him on a long road. Below was an English inscription: 'Be with us oh Lord for it is coming the dark.' The syntax stumbling toward that final word. Dark. Dante wears a long red robe, he is cloaked in the colour of human life. In another part of Florence I followed a sign that read DANTE'S CHURCH. Inside, beside the altar, was a piano with a burry tone. Someone played Bach, then Mozart, music which seemed right, part of the general blur of cultural brilliance, part of the grandeur of the past. But it would have been strange to Dante himself, born centuries before both those composers.

Dante was a soldier and a politician, and when his faction lost power he was expelled from the city. In exile, he was comforted by the sight of the sky; the most bitter political dispute could not deny him this vision. 'Can I not everywhere gaze upon the sun and stars?' He never returned to his place of birth, and is buried in Ravenna.

While in exile he wrote his great poem about the afterlife, filling it with enemies and friends, and at the heart of it he placed a woman, Beatrice, who is his guide in heaven. Beatrice was real. She lived, she met Dante when they were children, and years later was walking with friends in the streets of Florence when Dante saw her and slipped into rapture at the sound of her voice. She died in her twenties; the memory of her consumed the poet.

Is she like the watercolour girl? Laid out under glass above the bed of a man in love with books? I don't think so. *The Divine Comedy* depends on Beatrice moving about, being adored and talkative, determined.

Dante turned himself into a pilgrim in *The Divine Comedy*, making his way, with the help of the Roman poet Virgil and later Beatrice herself, from hell through purgatory to paradise. In *Paradise*, Dante asks Beatrice what causes the shadows on the moon. Are they the image of the banished Cain, carrying a bundle of thorns or briars from the spot where he killed his brother?

This story was a piece of folklore, told perhaps to children in Dante's time. Cain, the first murderer, had his face marked to protect him in some mysterious way from strangers who might kill him as he wandered in the exile that God decreed. Screen him up on the moon and he reminds everyone of sin, and of the possibility of compassionate protection, even if it is a grim, disfiguring one.

Beatrice corrects Dante. The shadows on the moon have nothing to do with sin and punishment. They're caused by the fact that the matter of the universe does not absorb God's grace equally; the moon is luminous but mottled, like unevenly dyed cloth.

Samuel Beckett, who was born in 1906, visited Florence for the first time when he was twenty-two. He had studied languages and knew his Dante. The young Beckett was a fine poet and an often anguished man; he moved between Paris, Germany, Dublin and London in a state of intermittent breakdown.

In wartime Paris he was a member of the Resistance, although he could have lived safely in Ireland. Like Dante, he chose exile. After his Resistance cell was exposed he was forced into hiding in the French countryside, and when he finally returned to Paris he lived in poverty and simplicity. Eventually he wrote novels that are like the long surge of a deeply confident mind.

Malone Dies is one of them. In it, Malone watches the moon through his window. Moonlight, it seems, is important to him – he tells us that he's afraid of the dark. 'A little darkness, in itself, at the time is nothing. You think no more about it and you go on. But I know what darkness is, it accumulates, thickens, then suddenly bursts and drowns everything.' For me, complete darkness is like the black floodwater of my childhood; a bad memory, a nightmare. Malone briefly wishes himself on the moon, dead, on that white and distant lifeless surface.

But in other passages Malone's moon is deeply human. Its shadows are the thorns carried by Cain, the image of slaughter and exile. Malone, too, knows his Dante, and he prefers the folk tale to Beatrice's theology of grace and receptivity, because there's no story there. No tale of the murder of a mild brother, the hot blight of guilt, and divine punishment. It's more consoling to live and die beneath a story, especially one telling of human impulsiveness and suffering, of harsh burdens and strange protection.

There's something else in all of this which speaks to me. Lines of reading join us across the vastness of time and place and language, like the lines drawn since ancient times by astronomers on the night sky, tracing the shapes of the constellations. I can lie in a hospital bed remembering a lost child in ancient Japan. In Beckett's short story 'Dante and the Lobster', his character holds an open copy of *The Divine Comedy*. 'He scooped his fingers under the book and shovelled it back till it lay wholly on his palms.' There: you have the weight, the pure pressure, of Dante's poem received in the hands.

Beckett read Dante, Dante was guided by the poet Virgil. In death they're forever linked by those who continue to read them. Time and place and differences in language recede, lovely and distant as an inky night, and our eyes also draw connections with other readers before us, even though they too, like the most remote of stars, may already be dead.

In that Florentine hotel room with shuttered windows near

the Medici Chapel, I had lilacs, marzipan, solitude. I read an English newspaper in the morning, before the scooters arrived on the streets. From first light, the shadows of pigeons moved swiftly through the room. The birds flew at my window, swerving up to the rooftop at the last moment, and I'd see a belly and claws, triangles of light feathers under the wings. The air glittered with their down, and with insects, leading the eye higher, away from the streets and squares into the sky.

'Can I not everywhere gaze on the sun and stars?' asks Dante, exiled from his city, knowing that his life would end in a strange place. Centuries on, Malone gazes at the moon from his deathbed. As a reader I contain them both. They and other writers are the constancies in my exile from the place of health, which I had always thought of as my rightful home. They are points of familiarity and reassurance in whatever place I lie.

Following the surgery to remove the cancer, I had six weeks to regain my strength for chemotherapy. Mothers Day came and went, and while the celebrations made me thankful for my survival, they also filled me with sadness. Chemotherapy would destroy my fertility, and although I was in my forties I had dreams of a late baby. I was frightened of the treatment for another reason too: a man I knew and liked had died of leukaemia just after my surgery. His chemotherapy had ravaged him swiftly, and it didn't work. It was a bad precedent for me.

The tests I underwent to determine heart, kidney and bone strength also felt ominous. Would my heart be at risk from this medicine? I was still tired from the after-effects of surgery and I was physically restricted; any expansion of my ribcage made the surgical incisions hurt. My normal solution in times of stress or difficulty – hard exercise – was impossible. If I breathed deeply I was in pain.

I got about in a state of false optimism, a survivor's euphoria that felt genuine at the time but was untrustworthy. Paradoxically I was also repeatedly, unexpectedly flooded with weakness and dread, as if I'd been given an intravenous sedative that wholly exhausted me. When this happened I was truly downcast; I would stare numbly at the floor, under the influence of some childish impression that if I kept still and self-contained I would be safe. It became a habit when I was alone: looking at nothing, looking down.

I saw a good deal of my GP. I didn't need to make appointments – his receptionist would lead me to a side room and he'd come to see me between his other patients. His diagnosis was simple and he repeated it kindly: I was experiencing grief, he explained. I knew, rationally, that I was devastated, I just didn't expect it to affect my body in this way. He always walked me to the door afterwards.

Later I would forget his explanation, I would be bewildered by my feelings and go back yet again to be calmed, to be cured of my transitory emotional paralysis. I am a tall woman but my GP is even taller, and I have to look up when I talk to him. I would raise my eyes and look about at his cheerful room, the bright curtains, at this substantial man who had swum the English Channel in a relay with six of his siblings to raise money for cancer research.

'You know you're going to make it,' he would say to me, every time. He freed me to look at the sky.

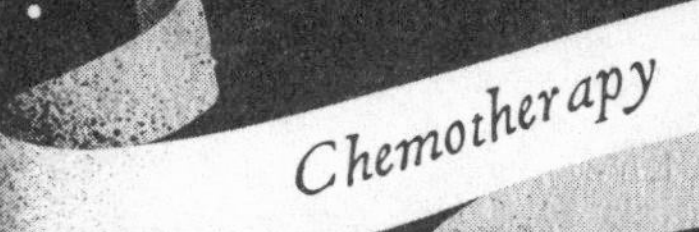
Chemotherapy

I have a taste for cold weather. That's easy to say when you live as I do in a warm seaside city, but I like the way the face numbs in severe Northern Hemisphere cold, the way a coat blows open in the wind. The exhilarating bite of the air, the possibility of snow. Snow changes everything. The air warms beforehand – and afterwards, if the fall is heavy enough, even a great city can almost be hushed.

A New York winter some twelve years ago gave me a passion for the cold. The whole city was white and silver and watercolour-brown. Lean squirrels rushed and paused, rushed and paused, over crusts of old snow. Cigar smoke seemed to pool and remain in the air, and I walked through these pools of smoky masculine breath long after the men who made them had ducked inside.

Chemotherapy is a little like a private winter. It brings its own weather, independent of the clouds or sunshine outside the hospital. But not all winters are pleasurable, full of interesting scenes for the traveller – some are simply bitter. During treatment, teeth chatter, sound travels differently, and the body must learn to wait, to endure. It's an icy climate, chemotherapy, and it's difficult to carry a living story out of that grey place, to set it down in light and warmth and hope it might hold together.

By the time I'd had my fourth episode of chemotherapy I'd lost my hair and my illness was visible and public. During my recovery from surgery the seriousness of my medical situation could be concealed, but twelve weeks on I was unmistakably suffering from cancer. In the oncologist's waiting room, many of us were as bald as monks and we felt a particular kinship, a solidarity that set us apart from the newly diagnosed and from those who had finished their treatment and were there for a check-up. Our faces were pale, with none of the fine surface hair that is unnoticed until it's gone. Light fell with strange clarity on our bare flesh, and this light seemed oddly familiar to me. Then I remembered the distinctness of women's eyelids in portraits by Jan van Eyck, and suddenly, even though we all looked deathly ill, we seemed to carry a Flemish light within us, something foreign, northern, bare and bright and cold, something deeply out of place in Australia. In the street, people stared; we were so thin we were almost fashionable, in a corpse-bride kind of way.

I had the first chemotherapy episode in an outpatients ward: a room with polished wooden flooring and tall windows overlooking a park. There were vast, end-of-the-day armchairs, fresh cake and chicken sandwiches, but no books or TV. It was companionable. Young men with younger wives at their sides boasted about the size of their tumours. At this stage I was curious as well as nervous, I noticed everything. The slide of the cannula into my vein. The machine that delivered the drugs, which made a fluttering noise like the wings of waterbirds striking the surface of a lake at take-off. I felt fine. Then I was seized with cold, my hearing dimmed, the ordinary world receded. Or it came in close, and this closeness felt dangerous. A few hours later, I started to be sick.

As I worked my way through the six treatments, I grew familiar with these symptoms, which were accompanied by an odd sense of paranoia. This seems to be common. I heard a singer who once had cancer describe how she expected to die every time the cannula was settled in her arm, every time the drugs began to thread through the plastic tubing. And I've read one perfect brief description of the effects of chemotherapy, by the American writer Joyce Wadler: 'I feel thick-headed, as if someone has hit me on the head with a sledge-hammer wrapped in a towel, but at the same time I'm anxious and speedy.'

Wadler describes the strange mixture of overexcitement and flat depression, the dull and jittery mood, the bad sleep. Everyone knows about hair loss and nausea, but mouth ulcers? A shredding of the walls of the tongue, making speech difficult?

I was so sick after my first treatment that I stayed overnight in hospital for the next five, while the fluttery machine washed saline through my veins. Someone came with a big silver space blanket when my teeth started to chatter. This was the pattern: one night in hospital, three weeks to recover, then a resigned return. I felt, childishly, that I was paying a terrible price for recovery. I felt that I was being punished.

My travel bag, the one with the space for a book under the zip, was starting to look rubbed around the edges, like the bag of a politician with a country constituency, or a mine worker on a fly-in, fly-out contract. One of the books I took to my chemo treatments was Alan Hollinghurst's *The Line of Beauty*, a novel strong enough to hold the attention of a person sitting upright in a hospital bed, waiting for a difficult night to fall. For a night of this kind you need a populous, witty but serious book, like *The Line of Beauty*. A good-sized book, in terms of characters and pages, is what's required, since the night will be long and the book shouldn't end too soon.

Hollinghurst's novel takes us into a world you see on the front page of broadsheets and tabloids, the world of British politics, and shows the way the popular press deals with privacy, including the publication of a diagnosis of AIDS. A gay man living provisionally in the household of a conservative politician has a grim insight into death. 'He stared out of the window, and after a minute found Henry James's phrase about the death of

Poe peering back at him. What was it? *The extremity of personal absence had just overtaken him.* The words, which once sounded arch and even facetious, were suddenly terrible to him, capacious, wise, and hard. He understood for the first time that they'd been written by someone whose life had been walked through, time and again, by death.'

'Personal absence' is such an elegant, dispassionate way to describe death, but if you think about it, the phrase is crushingly extreme. And death – as distinct from fantasies of murder and criminal investigation – walked through the lives of people with much greater immediacy in the nineteenth century, when the dying were nursed at home. There was almost a cult of mourning: physical relics such as hair were commonly retained, sketches were sometimes made of the dead. The wearing of black for extended periods was ritually observed in well-ordered households.

In our times we tend to focus on aberrant death, the basis of so much of our entertainment. Not that this was absent in the nineteenth century; we are the inheritors of Poe's detective stories, the forerunners of the investigative dramas we enjoy now. Today, of course, we also have forensics, and the case-by-case resolution of individual deaths, creating the illusion that mortality is a problem that can be solved.

When I was very low – after the first few sessions of chemotherapy, after the routine was established but before the end was in sight – my high-school boyfriend tracked down my phone number and began to call from the other side of the country. His voice was a little indistinct but still recognisable, and suddenly I was fifteen again, filling a bucket with blackberries pulled from canes that bent over cold shallow water, or sitting on a gravestone in a country cemetery, wearing an op-shop dress while he took black and white photos with an important-looking camera. I was a long way from the hospital, wrapped in memory and a familiar voice.

How is it possible to submit to all this? To sit with the other Flemish faces in the oncologist's waiting room, to settle into a hospital bed with a book, then lay the book down to push up a sleeve when the nurse arrives with the drugs and the machine, and turn calmly aside? You need to have confidence in the medicine, but it's also possible because the mind turns everything into a story.

Each phone call from a friend, each medical visit reinforced this. 'How have you been?' the kind oncologist would ask casually, from behind her desk. And the previous three weeks of partial recovery – a lurid, shattered jumble of sudden shocks, unpleasant sensations and events – lined up neatly in the form of a story that someone else was listening to, with interest.

I wasn't a perfect patient. 'How can you do this?' I asked the oncologist before my fourth treatment. I was in the mood for complaint.

'I can do this,' she answered sensibly, 'because I'm going to save your life.'

The young men in the outpatients room made themselves heroes of tales of misdiagnosis or difficult surgery. They were happy because they had control of a story, and in a terrible way they were happy because they weren't about to run out of material, not yet, not with a cannula in their arm, different from every other cannula. There was the drama of insertion, and fresh dialogue with the nurse; they were amassing new material as they spoke.

What will happen next? we ask ourselves, often dreamily, all through our lives. Let's go to the hospital. Let's find out what happens next.

Nobody accepts that it might be death. In *Anna Karenina*, Anna's little son Seryozha is told that his mother is dead. It's a lie, and he protects himself from it in the only way he can. 'He did not believe in death generally, and in her death in particular . . .' He's right about his mother and he does see her, briefly, again, which must encourage his conviction. 'He did not believe that those he loved could die, above all that he himself could die.' We all have a little of Seryozha within us.

I have a postcard of Mt Fuji tucked in the back of a book. The mountain is photographed from an angle that renders it deep blue, almost the same colour as the sky. If it weren't for the snow it would be easy to mistake the slope of the mountain for a slight darkening of the sky. I read somewhere that when the

Europeans who first climbed Mt Fuji saw the view they forgot what it cost them to get to the top – some of them unlaced their boots to find that their toenails had floated off in little ponds of blood.

On the back of the postcard a Japanese woman I knew when I was a student has written: 'I'm going to be all right. I wish I could visit you.' I let myself believe, for a time, that she was going to survive advanced bone cancer.

When I was going through chemotherapy I felt that I wore my life lightly, and oddly enough this was a great relief. My life was charged with narrative meaning but it was also unimportant. I was thin, in more ways than one. I felt free to go. I didn't want to, I had my son and my work, but I felt that if I chose to loosen my grip on them I could easily slip away. It didn't necessarily feel sad.

Perhaps I'm romanticising this. Perhaps I spent too much of my adolescence sitting cross-legged on gravestones. But when I think of that time in treatment it has a wintry glitter; my face was like the face of a stranger in the mirror and I was strangely glad to be clear of my ordinary, comfortable self. What I didn't enjoy was the means of escape.

I would recover from the immediate effects of the drugs in about three days, after which I was filled with a sense of directionless urgency without being capable of accomplishing much, and this bewildered me. Lauren had to remind me I was seriously ill. 'You have to give in to your illness,' she said. But still I tried to rush about; I didn't *want* to understand.

Martin Amis has a short story, a parody of schoolboy composition, called 'What Happened to Me on Holiday'. It's about that moment in all our lives when the fact of death is suddenly, appallingly understood.

The narrator, a child, is on a seaside holiday with his brother when a family friend dies in London. The child registers the impact of Elias's death on the adults around him, including Elias's brother, who is also close to the child and his parents. The deep unease that comes with the awareness that a sibling can die, can be lost forever, is depicted as waking up to find the adjacent bed empty. It's an intense and domestic understanding of a brother's death. Life, it seems, is just a holiday from death, and death is imagined in terms of a lapse in water safety: Elias drowned while swimming, and to the child it's as if he forgot to wear his floaties, his 'armies'.

I remember blowing up yellow floaties when my son was learning to swim; every child in the pool was held up by a parent's breath trapped in quilted plastic. In his story, Amis is making a striking pun on the word 'armies'. When we die we go swimming without the armies of our friends, our families, our doctors;

we who were as mighty as great commanders, as generals with our troops, are suddenly, sinkingly, alone. To grow up is to put off your protection and to die. We all have to do this, although we postpone the final moment for as long as we can.

And, what's almost worse, we're aware that we will die and pass into the unknown, but we have to put this fact from our minds so we can get on with our ordinary lives. Until sickness, or another person's death, reminds us of the inevitability. The acknowledgement of death rises and subsides in us like waves that must be ridden out. We keep our heads above this dangerous water to avoid being submerged in fear, or in hopeless resignation.

Late in the sequence of my chemotherapy sessions, I heard another story about drowning from a nun called Sister Rita, who was sharing my hospital room. It's a story about survival, too, and it kept me afloat like buoyant timber in the aftermath of a shipwreck.

Sister Rita's story could have come from the nineteenth century, when nuns and shipwrecks were among the staples of popular Gothic fiction. (Poe's brother Henry wrote one of these tales, but a modern hospital is not a setting that Poe's brother could have easily imagined.)

How odd it is to lie in the same room as a stranger. Whole families appear at hospital bedsides and speak unguardedly about their love. Angry patients spread their belongings all over the room and call the nurses to complain about nothing. Someone's favourite television show blares out. But if you're lucky you get a room where everyone is considerate, and when the visitors leave there's the companionability of small talk and, finally, sleep.

One night Sister Rita, whose medical treatment didn't involve chemotherapy, was lying in the bed next to mine. We talked for a time and I discovered that we were almost neighbours – her convent was at the end of my street. I was hooked up to the machine that sounded like birds' wings. There was always a delay between the delivery of drugs into my circulation and the onset of the worst side-effects. Late in the night, when I was very sick, Sister Rita came to my bedside in her blue pyjamas and held my hands. When she released them she made the sign of the cross on my forehead with a practised thumb. I was grateful for her faith, although I don't share or understand it.

Then she sat on the side of my bed and told me her story. She had joined her order in Cork, although her mother was against it. 'Have you had enough yet?' she would ask whenever Rita went home. At twenty, Sister Rita left Ireland, travelling with another young nun across the world to teach Polish, Yugoslav and Aboriginal children in a mining town in Western Australia. She understood their struggles: her own language of preference was Irish, not English. She loved her work, she was happy, and then she was shipwrecked.

This is how it happened: a young priest organised an outing in a boat on a local estuary, for himself, the Mother Superior and the nuns. The light and space must have been so beautiful after the crowded classrooms in which they worked, but the boat capsized far from shore and everybody was lost except Sister Rita and her friend, who were carried out to the open sea. They couldn't swim.

The boat rolled in the swell and they grasped at the sliding hull until they found new and freshly agonising fingerholds. It grew dark; they watched through the night for the whiteness of water breaking in the distance, calling out to one another when each wave struck. All night they kept their weary, painful grip on the rim of the hull. Toward morning Sister Rita lost her strength. She called out to Jesus for what she thought was the last time, and then she heard the sound of fishing boats, coming to save them.

The next day the people of the town and their children came to the beach and found all those who'd been drowned and carried them back from the sand and the sea.

In my own terrible night Sister Rita told me to open my hands. She sprinkled my palms with Lourdes water.

'It will feel colder than any other kind of water,' she said. But she may as well have simply said, Hold on.

By the sixth treatment I was so frail I couldn't hide the anxiety in my voice when I phoned my mother from my hospital bed. She heard it and said, 'I'm coming, I'm coming right now.'

She had to drive a great distance in the early hours to an airport in northern New South Wales, wait for connections in other airports, stand in a queue at a taxi rank. But she flew across the country at a moment's notice because of something she sensed in my voice, despite my feigned strength and confidence. She brought money and books and she was as blunt and casual about it all as the oncologist. They had the same job. They were both saving my life.

When my son was a baby he slept badly. I used to wake in the night just before I heard him move or cry. A mother listens, does her sleepy, irritable, late-night diagnosis, and comes to a child's bedside in the dark, even when the child is a grown woman in a hospital bed on the other side of a vast desert.

I want to tell you a story about my mother. In midwinter of 2008, after all my medical treatment was finished, we went to Bali because I wanted to be in a warm place. Somewhere very different from the hospital rooms where I waited, had surgery or chemotherapy. The week before I flew to Denpasar, my son's grandmother died, on her ninety-second birthday – a few hours after the speeches honouring her life, after the grandchildren had packed away their guitars, after the leftover cake had been wrapped. She couldn't have planned it better.

At the funeral there was a basket of offerings: wheat stalks, eucalyptus leaves and roses. We filed to the coffin and chose our final gifts for her. Mine was wheat, the grains packed in tight rows, not a whisker out of place. I hoped they would burn with her when she was cremated; I hoped that wheat-smoke would rise above her ashes. As it happened, this ceremony was a precursor of a cremation procession my mother and I saw in Ubud.

Because everyone thinks of Bali as a kind of heaven, you arrive almost braced for disappointment. This dissolves when you see the temple carvings, the lotus ponds, the canvases of lotuses – which are disturbingly lovely, so strange and entertaining, so wholly fulfilling the task of art to loosen and stretch the real. Yet this isn't paradise. There are dogs with the dull coats of illness or malnutrition in the streets, women carrying loads of rice or even concrete on their heads; and the air in Ubud smells of benzine from the constant river of motorcycles.

There have been bombings down on the coast, and terrible executions.

Security men checked the underside of our car with mirrors when we arrived at the hotel. It wasn't an ordinary hotel, it was a line of thatched pavilions on a ridge above a watercourse, each one opening onto a garden. Offerings to the spirits were placed high and low: incense, rice on squares of palm leaves, woven platters heaped with flowers and crackers. Fear and protection were all around us; steps were being taken to fend off political and spiritual danger.

In Bali, the spirits of the dead are considered to be on the path to reincarnation, and funerals are not sombre. There's a fantastic involvement with human remains. The dead are first buried and then, in time, exhumed, washed and cremated. The bones are ground to pieces and cast into water, in order to be carried to the sea. For reincarnation to take place, something of the dead person must be in the earth, something must be in the air, and something in the water, or so we were told by our taxi driver, talking casually over his shoulder in the thick traffic of motorcycles and people.

At the funeral of H.G. Wells in London in 1946, a mourner accidentally bumped the button controlling the cremation mechanism, and Wells was carried away before the end of the ceremony. Such disruption to the sequence of prayer, procession and burning would put the Balinese spirit in jeopardy.

If the dead have been publicly important in Bali, their exhumed bodies are carried through the streets in a tower behind a fabulous carved effigy, before being cremated. My mother and I sat on a wall beside the pavement for hours to see the bull-shaped effigies and the towers that carried the bodies of a prince and a chief of police. A huge festive crowd waited with us; there were sarong-sellers and young boys whose T-shirts had been printed by someone who didn't read English, or who did, but in a way I didn't want to think about. Shirtless Westerners strolled past with locally done tattoos on display. People gathered at the very edge of rooftops.

The effigy and tower carriers, dressed in the black and white cloth that signifies the interweaving of good and evil, took up their positions and the procession began. We'd seen one of the effigies unexpectedly the previous day, an immense black bull moving haltingly along the streets as men with forked sticks lifted power lines high above its horns. Workers were fitting teeth to the demons on a tower.

Both bulls and towers were spectacular, and we had only the most basic idea of what they meant. How potent they must be to people who live by their significance. They were carried in turns by hundreds of men, who had to set them down after only a short distance, their strength exhausted, for a fresh group to step forward. This dipping and rising motion, the swift, staggering rush and sudden arrest of progress, made the weight visible, muscular, humanly important. It also made the streets dangerous; the throng was so tightly packed against the buildings lining the road that the carriers could not avoid collisions, even trampling.

Men who were balanced on a crowded wall helped my mother to safety. How small she was. Delicate and silver-haired, she reached only to the shoulders of the Balinese. After the procession had passed and she climbed down, I made a barrier around her with my arms; she seemed not to notice what I was trying to do.

We didn't go to the cremation ceremony at the temple, where an even denser crowd had formed, and instead walked out of town on a road filled with slow-moving motorcycles and tired families. Should we stop and wait until the traffic cleared? I imagined a tyre bumping her, a fall. Surely she too was afraid?

But she wouldn't stop. At the gates of our hotel she turned to me and smiled. 'See?' she said. 'I brought you safely home.'

We watched the cremation on television. Flame poured from the ears and mouths of the bulls, whose job it was to carry the spirits of the dead to safety. The following night, when the wind blew in our direction, the air was full of ash.

A day or so later, watching a display of trained elephants in a mountain reserve, I saw my mother betray the fear she'd been too proud to show at the cremation. The elephants had to walk along a log at some height from the ground, clasping one another's tails in their trunks, then climb down on timber stepping-stones. When they tested a step before trusting their weight to it, my mother turned away in sympathy. She too knew the fear of falling.

And something else: she was still, in her mind, the mother, the big animal who would transport her child home.

I was so sorry for the way I'd disrupted her life. She had her own books to write, her own household, her throng of grandchildren. When she arrived at my hospital bed after the sixth, most devastating chemotherapy treatment, I tried to apologise. But she brushed aside my words. 'I was feeling my age,' she said. 'Then you got sick and I had to act, and I knew I wasn't old.'

In the three-week breaks between chemotherapy sessions, I spent a lot of time in a car park above the beach near my house, looking out through the windscreen at the winter ocean, milky with froth and sand, at waves chopping across one another in stormy disorder. In the early mornings, before work, I liked to walk along the river. I'd rest on a park bench looking down on the water, the boats, and the sand-spit where lovers go, I'm told, on moonless nights. Imagine. The sand no wider than a child's bed. Someone had taped a message to one of the benches asking a woman to forgive him, and to phone. It stayed there through the whole winter.

The park was near Sister Rita's convent. I called in to see her on one of my walks, and she gave me a quick tour. 'This is how we bless ourselves,' she said, making the sign of the cross as we were leaving the chapel. Salvation may come from a mysterious spiritual height, or it may come from our own fingers, dipped in holy water, holding onto the rim of an upturned boat in the ocean.

The critic James Wood, like my grandmother, feels free to discuss the human soul. He tracks the history of stream of consciousness, that literary style whereby the movement of the mind is set down in such a way as to raise the novel above simple description. Wood calls it 'the soul's stutter'. When we read it we are with another person more closely than if we were in love. We believe in these characters, yet we also understand that they do not exist. We're at once alone and in close company: this is the great gift of the novel, the element that makes reading more than a solitary pastime. We sit within another's person.

James Wood traces stream of consciousness back to soliloquy, that point in a drama where an actor steps forward and offers their thoughts to the obscure faces beyond the stage lights. And he traces soliloquy to prayer. As readers we listen, an invisible audience in a theatre where it matters, deeply, almost religiously, to speak and to be heard.

During chemotherapy, sound seemed oddly muffled. My eyesight, too, would dim from time to time, then quickly right itself. This was not dangerous, I was told – it was a temporary vascular problem, like migraine – but it frightened me. What if my sight were to fail entirely? How could I live without a free and impulsive choice of books? How limiting would Braille be?

If I became blind, would I be lonely, banished to the social world of conversation with real people instead of communing with characters in novels? And if I were to use audio books, would the company of characters imagined by me when alone be lost? Would the inflection of an actor's voice deny me that deep interior closeness of the soul?

Once chemotherapy was over, I came to trust that my vision would return to normal, to believe the diagnosis and wait out the time it took for my sight to clear. My hearing, too, stabilised, but the changes in my senses unnerved me. The ear itself, which functions physiologically to maintain balance, has quite a part to play also in terror and instability, something Poe well knew.

Ask an older person, someone over eighty, about Edgar Allan Poe. Mention 'The Pit and the Pendulum'. They'll remember the story and the schoolroom where it was read to them, and the bed they went home to, and the struggle to stay awake in case the forces of the Spanish Inquisition rose up to stage a late, mad attack on the weak and helpless heretics of Australia.

Nobody forgets a Poe story. They take us back to a time when libraries felt spooky, and sensational tales seeped into the bodies of susceptible readers, speeding up the heartbeat, creating a physical impatience if, for some reason, you had to lay the book aside. This can still happen now: it helps if you read by lamplight. It helps if the space beyond the light is busy with shadow.

My school library seemed to belong to the time of reading by lamp or candlelight, and was a spooky place. Nobody culled the books. The shelves were packed with classics and curiosities. Here you could read Churchill's speeches, or a translation of *À Rebours*, the once notorious French novel that Oscar Wilde was questioned about in the trial that resulted in his imprisonment. Dickens and the Russians were there in the library, and Zola, Emily Dickinson, Patrick White, Homer, Byron. Japanese poetry on foxed pages. Poe too, although I didn't read him then. And it was in the school library that I first saw photos of the Holocaust, the death camps: the evidence of real horror.

A famous Old Boy had sent the library the head of a mummy. He was an anatomist who had the task of excavating graves in Egypt before their contents were lost under the Aswan Dam, so he had plenty of mummies to hand. Ours was a young girl; someone had snapped her head off and left her body behind. The neck was glued to the bottom of a glass box on a table, so that she was displayed at student height. Her skin was tarry, her teeth like chalk; she had stiff, crumpled eyelids, and reddish hair poking through the tar.

For the most part it was easy to forget that she'd been human, except for her hair. That was real, just like our own. The hands that had tended this hair were lost in Egypt; the mummy's eyes were lost too, as was her skin. But her hair was with us and it made her something more than hard old flesh and teeth. It made her sad, and human.

The town itself wasn't exactly neutral in the matter of spookiness. It was built on the banks of a wide flooding river, under a sky that flocked with fruit bats at twilight. There was even a castle, a crenellated mansion, further upriver.

When I was a child I found a baby bat in the school grounds. He had dropped from the electrocuted body of his mother, which was still gripping the power lines that killed her. I remember the scrabble of his hooks on my bare hands, his orphan desperation. He didn't survive long. To me, he was an infant being with eyes the colour of shallow river water, but other people see bats differently. The English scientist Francis Ratcliffe 'had to fight back an uneasy desire for sunlight and human company' when he dealt with them. In the daytime they sleep folded in their wings in favourite trees, in big stinking colonies, each one wrapped like a secret. They don't fly in daylight; I never saw one flap past the library window, past the glass case of the mummy.

Poe wrote a story called 'Some words with a Mummy'. After Poe died and was buried his body was exhumed, and there is a gruesome account of the state of his remains. The sexton who lifted the skull heard a thud when he shifted the thing. The brain had dried and it fell from side to side, he said, just like a lump of mud. It's a macabre detail, idly memorable. Poe's true remains are thudding away not in the soil of Virginia but on the page, where his words touch a common pulse; our own blood beats in our ears as we read.

'The Tell-Tale Heart' is Poe's story about a murderer making his confession to the unsuspecting police. He does this because he thinks he hears the heartbeat of his victim, stowed under the floorboards of the room where the police are conducting their interview. Haunted by hallucination, guilty, sick with terror, he betrays himself.

There's no narrative distance in this story. The storyteller jabs a finger at you, the reader; he comes at you like something fighting to break out of the floor under your chair. 'True! – nervous – very, very dreadfully nervous I have been and am; but why *will* you say that I am mad? The disease had sharpened my senses – not destroyed – not dulled them. Above all was the sense of hearing acute. I heard all things in the heaven and in the earth. I heard many things in hell. How, then, am I mad? Hearken! And observe how healthily – how calmly I can tell you the whole story.'

These opening lines are an accusation, and as I read I'm taking them personally: I've been cast in the role of an accuser, or a medical authority, diagnosing insanity. The narrator is arguing against such a diagnosis. He thinks, wrongly, he can tell a story calmly, so he must be healthy. Freud assessed his patients in the same way; if you gave a coherent account of yourself, he looked for physical disease instead of hysteria. What has happened in the darkened room of 'The Tell-Tale Heart'? What has caused a man to be reduced to this level of jittery but articulate delusion? As imaginary doctor, as analyst, as reader, I must know.

The victim is an old man who trusts his murderer. The murderer in turn loves his victim, even as he begins to develop an aggressive phobia about the old man's eye, which has a white membrane across the cornea. It reminds the murderer, unreasonably, of the eye of a vulture and so the old man must be destroyed.

Nightly the murderer checks his victim. The eyes are closed, there is nothing offensive about the sleeping man, he's permitted to live – until the moment when the attacker shines a light on the face of the wakeful old man and sees again the appalling eye. He kills the old man, cuts him up, thrusts him into the space below the floor.

All seems innocent to the police, seated above the evidence of the crime. Then the murderer hears the pulse of the dead heart under the floorboards, and his confident story collapses into the criminal truth, into a halting and jagged confession demonstrating both madness and culpability. All because of something he thought he heard.

Sound is fundamental to the lives of most of us. Hearing brings us music, and music can wholly shift a state of mind. Perhaps it can shift the state of mind of a whole population, or at least a generation. The composer George Antheil saw a kind of physical salvation in post-war jazz, which, he wrote, 'made us remember at least that we still had bodies which had not been exploded by shrapnel'. We can fall in love with a voice, as Dante did, on a street in Florence when Beatrice spoke and his long adoration began. How porous we all are; how susceptible sound makes us, to happiness or terror. How hard it is, for a person with good hearing, to imagine living without sound.

The South African poet David Wright, in a moving account of deafness, writes that 'the deaf do not, because they cannot, deal in the nuances – particularly the verbal nuances – of personal relations. Their dealings are direct – may appear outrageously direct; their handshakes are ungloved.' Nuance: so important in life as well as in art.

And the deaf seem to attract peculiar, inaccurate projections; other people misread them. In Joseph Conrad's *Under Western Eyes* the hero's eardrums are burst, deliberately, in a cold and savage attack. Suddenly his world is silent. He lies in shock and pain on the street. 'Silent men, moving unheard, lifted him up, laid him on the sidewalk, gesticulating and grimacing around him their alarm, horror and compassion. A red face with moustaches stooped close over him, lips moving, eyes rolling.' Compassion can't break through the silence. Without the sound of their voices his rescuers seem to be hamming it up, acting out an exaggerated and unconvincing concern. The injured man creates a false impression. His shocked face appears to be 'composed in meditation', his bewilderment is read as serenity.

After I lost my hair, after I became so very thin, I became the target of curious stares and I had to learn to feign serenity as a method of self-protection. I felt the sick fear of anyone who has experienced a great disturbance in their senses. I felt the Gothic, the unsettled and the extreme within myself, and I wondered if these changes would be permanent.

In Gothic fiction, characters must contend with the dead, with active hauntings or with hallucinations of hauntings, as well as whatever other trying circumstances they might find themselves in: orphanhood, lunacy, imprisonment, inheritances that go astray, troubling romantic situations. The Gothic novel does not strive for subtlety, and it isn't to everyone's taste. It can seem adolescent, an immature version of the stately, measured, grown-up realist novel, except that the line between the Gothic and the realist is never clear. A disdain for the Gothic is limiting, since this literature, in all its flagrancy, has something to say about emotional as well as physical death, and a tale of a haunting can have a narrative vitality that is far from conclusive. Gothic stories linger especially in the mind.

Donna Tartt's novel *The Secret History* needs to be read with, or after, Poe. Like 'The Tell-Tale Heart', it opens with a confession. In unflaggingly relaxed and elegant language Richard Papen begins his story of a murder he helped organise. Richard is an outsider – Californian, poor, in a circle of spoiled and patrician classics students at a small university in Vermont. The university aims, according to its advertising material, to inculcate the civilising effects of culture, but in fact it has the usual campus mixture of drugs and alcohol, loud music, bad art, pompous and exclusive staff, unhappy sex, scorned subgroups, snobs, and intelligent adolescent capability – the kind that can organise a murder.

Had there been no murder, *The Secret History* would be a deeply funny campus novel. Had the murder been less deftly handled, it would be a good mystery novel, in a shrewdly observed setting. But it's more than this. Tartt writes about our uneasy relationship with ourselves. About how we might, in seeking some temporary reprieve from ourselves, precipitate a situation, a mood, an acute and intolerable frame of mind, which can never be reversed.

Six classics students – Francis, Henry, Bunny, twins Charles and Camilla, and Richard – meet at a country mansion belonging to Francis' aunt. It should be haunted but it isn't. There are dust sheets and a distant caretaker, dim corridors, a spiky roof. A photo, in the family gallery, of a great-uncle who drowned on the *Titanic*, and a grand library with a chandelier, a monstrous fireplace, and a piano where Charles, half drunk, plays Chopin. There's a mordant humour in all this: Richard is told that the great-uncle's tennis racquet was found floating above the shipwreck, as if the man went under mid-serve, leaving a buoyant tombstone.

In the mansion the group make plans to recreate the conditions of the Bacchanalia – the delirium of violence and ecstasy familiar from their study of ancient Greek. Why? Henry explains it to Richard, who is a latecomer to the experiment: 'one mustn't underestimate the primal appeal – to lose one's self, lose it utterly'. It's a more referenced, more ironically civilised and dangerous version of standard student alcoholic excess. It leads to hallucinatory destruction and then, as part of a cover-up, to clear-headed murder. The murderers escape conviction but they don't go unpunished. The self is indeed lost.

In the aftermath of the carnage, Richard suffers from a kind of dissociation: 'White sky. Trees fading at the skyline, the mountains gone. My hands dangled from the cuffs of my jacket as if they weren't my own.' You feel his state, in the blurted sentences.

Like the murderer in 'The Tell-Tale Heart', Richard is obsessed with palpitation. 'The objects in the room seemed to swell and recede with each thump of my heart. In a horrible daze, I sat on my bed, one elbow on the windowsill, and tried to pull myself together.' He fears his heart will burst. Until finally, even this intensity is lost. 'I lay on my bed. I felt my heart limping in my chest, and was revolted by it, a pitiful muscle, sick and bloody, pulsing against my ribs.'

He is estranged from his heart, which speaks for all his panic and entrapment. Richard is the victim under the floorboards with the impossibly amplified heart; he is the unhappy and confessional murderer, and he will never be the same again.

Is it possible to lose yourself safely, retrievably? To step outside yourself and, more importantly, when you've had enough, step back in? At one point in *The Secret History*, Henry offers this insight into reading: 'if one is to read Dante, and understand him, one must become a Christian if only for a few hours'. A kind of method acting for the reader. I don't think he's right, exactly. I don't think it can be done. You can't take a quick dip in Christianity, or any other religion. But reading *is* a temporary loosening of the ego. How else are we able to imagine Richard's plight, to pity him, to lay aside our condemnation of his acts? When we read we move away from ourselves. We listen without the vulnerable physiology of the human ear. We dissolve, just a little; we're pleasurably lost. Then, in a few hours, we close the book and we're home again, and this is welcome, even if the home of the self is poisoned, sick with difficult drugs and strangely lit.

There's an Irish folktale about an old woman who, at the end of an eventful life, decides to go back to the convent she ran away from as a girl. She expects to have to explain herself to the nuns who have lived their peaceful routine lives within the convent walls, but in fact nobody noticed she was gone. The Virgin Mary has disguised herself as the wayward nun and performed all her duties in the time she's been away.

There are times, now that my medical treatment is over, when I'd like to pretend that something like this happened to me. Someone else, with my name, with a son and a job like mine, went through the cancer treatment in my place. But then I'm reminded of what I would lose if I were to disown my experience in such a way: the understanding that my life has shape and urgency, as well as everyday routine; the awareness that my own and others' lives compose themselves in narrative, especially when in jeopardy.

Those years of cancer showed me that although all of us have times when the self might weigh heavily – as it can even in its ordinary familiarity, let alone in pain and anxiety – when we long to be someone else, somewhere else, it's not estrangement from ourselves we yearn for, so much as a release into the account of another's life. A release in extended storytelling.

It was a particularly bad time for me to be sick. For five years I'd been writing *The Wing of Night*, a novel about the First World War. In those days I had an overriding taste for stark emotional truth: I thought this was the first job of the novelist, and I wanted to get some sense of the permanent mental wreckage of great terror, of fear that refuses to simply go away once a place of safety is reached. Fear that metastasises into hallucination, confusion, sometimes violence.

Now I have other concerns. Illness has made me consider what might be redemptive, and to value, deeply, the fact that the most devastated lives are surely also touched, if only briefly, with a remitting hopeful sense of purpose. Sometimes, in places where ill people gather – waiting rooms, a chemotherapy ward – this purpose is concentrated on personal narrative, on the ordinary task of telling a neighbour a story, and the act itself is charged with life, even though the story may concern the end of it.

The impulse to write *The Wing of Night* was deeply grounded in my reading, and also in my childhood. My paternal grandfather was at Gallipoli, before being shot in France. He wasn't at the original landing; he arrived in September and was there for the blizzards that froze men at their posts. He was an orphan and a farm boy, and judging by his medical records his teeth hurt. He died before I was born, but I met him in my grandmother's stories, in the house he built, where I spent my childhood, and in a particular book: a volume of the *Official History of Australia in the War of 1914–18*, which falls open most easily at views of a desolate French landscape destroyed by the battle of Pozières. He must have looked at those pages repeatedly.

When he came back to Australia, my grandfather built the timber house I lived in as a child, but he wasn't able to put the war behind him. The house had wide silver verandahs and a garden full of mangoes, peaches and pecans. It was a paradise for a child, but it wasn't always sunny. The family stories, told over sugared tea, were often about war. I like to think that he imagined all his grandchildren when he built the sad and beautiful spaces of his house, as intensely as I imagined him when I wrote my novel. I wanted to write about poor boys with great imaginations, I didn't want to write about the battle manoeuvres of soldiers.

But this came at a price. Readers complained, quite rightly, about the sadness. 'You withdraw every consolation you advance,' said one of my bright and honest students on reading the book.

Saul Bellow once talked about writing a book so miserable that he would have been better off apprenticing himself to an undertaker. At a time when I was a little too close to the undertakers for comfort, I had to sell a vigorously disconsolate novel. I was bald and thin after four sessions of chemotherapy, I couldn't hear very well and my voice was whispery. Around my medical schedule and work at the university, I did publicity photos, interviews, attended festivals. The publication of a book would normally be a nail-biting time when I worried about its reception, but because my nails were already bitten to the quick, as it were, I was free, in a strange way, to enjoy myself.

Festivals often have sessions called 'Meet the Writer', which are also about a writer meeting readers – a great experience from my point of view. All that silent writing, all that hushed reading can turn into talk and laughter and good wine, and the spillage of personality outside the pages. Here – this is what we look like, we readers, we writers, meeting at last like big families parted generations ago through accident or immigration, now hoping to find resemblances, or debate, in a break from an otherwise ordinary week.

And festivals require writers to travel, to get out from behind their desks and move around in the world of flight schedules and hotel rooms – professionally interesting places, aeroplanes and strange rooms being the habitats of reading and stories.

Travel is also the traditional privilege of certain illnesses. In *Illness as Metaphor*, Susan Sontag quotes two great writers, each suffering from tuberculosis. Here is Robert Louis Stevenson: 'By a curious irony, the places to which we are sent when health deserts us are often singularly beautiful . . .' And Katherine Mansfield: 'I seem to spend half of my life arriving at strange hotels . . .' Writers' festivals had handed me something like the popular nineteenth-century remedy for tuberculosis. I was going to see the world, or at least a few cities. Strange hotels were making up beds for me.

The first hotel had brown furniture and a tartan wallpaper border just below the cornice. A friend, Anita, flew in to keep an eye on me; I didn't mention how badly I needed her company, I didn't have to tell her how very grateful I was. Soon the room was brimming with our suitcases and shoes. We talked for a while after we switched out the lights, and she told me the story of how she came to be there, drifting off to sleep in her husband's comforting pyjamas.

Her parents had had an arranged marriage. They met just before the wedding when her father travelled from Guangzhou to Sydney. He was supposed to marry Anita's aunt but she bluntly refused him, and a younger, more dutiful sister, Anita's mother, was laced into the wedding dress instead. Was there a common language between bride and groom? Shared customs? Happiness? Or just the need to bear the designated grandchildren?

We talked some more, then agreed to go to sleep, but the story of Anita's parents rose to the ceiling, it pressed against the wallpaper. I was distracted from my own anxieties by the dutiful self-discipline of that Chinese bride.

The next hotel had a vast bath surrounded by marble and I was quite alone. I floated, added more hot water, floated some more, recalling a phrase from *Henry IV*: 'out of this nettle, danger, men pluck this flower, safety'. Repeating it and taking comfort in the rhythm, which works like a mathematical equation: if this (danger), then this (safety).

I arrived at the third hotel at twilight. The room was spectacular: walls of glass which could be closed off in sections with wooden shutters in a game of make-your-own-window. Outside, there was a translucent sunny haze, as if the air had decided to hold onto the last of the light. The remnants of a colonial city lay far below: straight streets and modest Victorian domes.

In the morning, hot-air balloons floated past, rendering the sky orderly and composed. Later came the sound of church bells, and when I got up and looked down at the steps of the cathedral I saw a little pond of white: a bride. She might have been gritting her teeth but she wasn't, at that moment, running away, although I felt that she was quite free to do so if she chose. I spread the city's newspaper across the bed and began to read.

Elsewhere I had less happy experiences: places with telephones that didn't work, rooms that stank of cigarette smoke and garbage bins, unwiped circles from other people's coffee cups all over the bedside table. I killed cockroaches with a laminated welcome card and worried about my low immunity to disease.

Something tangible sits on my long white writing table to remind me of this time. When checking in at a hotel for one literary event I was handed a box, a gift from the organisers. Other writers were opening their own boxes in the lobby behind me. We'd been given paperweights, poured by some trick of the glassblower into a shape that exactly fitted the human palm. It had the quality of an ancient implement, something smoothed by human effort, an object vital to survival. I could have slept with it in my hand. We all compared them in the lobby; there were various colours but mine was an intense blue, the colour you sometimes see when you look out the window of an aeroplane and realise that you're flying into dawn.

The last hotel was in the countryside in England, outside Cheltenham. Elizabethan with a Victorian overlay. In the garden an ammonite fossil was balanced on a stone post beside a flight of steps, as if some whiskery Darwinist had just put down his hammer and chisel and gone indoors for tea.

In my room I lay in bed under a huge beam and tried to take stock of my life. Months had passed since the release of my book, and I had finished chemotherapy, but I had become superstitious; I looked for symbols everywhere, like a schoolgirl writing an essay on a difficult poem. What could the leaded windows mean? The gunshots from the meadows in the distance? I raised the sheet protectively over myself. It was going to be a long flight home.

The oddest room I've ever stayed in was in New York, one summer before my illness was diagnosed, when I was trying to think of reasons for my exhaustion – work, jetlag – not yet knowing it was due to cancer. (My surgeon later estimated that the cancer had begun around this time.) I was staying in a hostel that had been established for poor immigrants, and I slept, as they must have done, in a single bed with a plain wooden cross hanging above my pillow. My window overlooked another room, which was empty, and through the filmy glass I could see a shadowy Jesus in red and cream robes carrying a child.

In the morning two men clumped about on a ledge outside. I heard them discussing the state of the building, saying it wasn't sound, that the wall behind my head took the full force of storms. Even from inside, the walls looked brittle; they were textured with scraped plaster, paint that was crazed and lifting. Cardboard was taped over a hole opposite the lifts, and the lights were dim. But the courtyard under my window was thick with azaleas, the kitchen served fresh cherry bread, and I decided that the old walls were strong enough to stay upright for the few nights I was sleeping there, on my way to visit a friend in upstate New York.

This friend owned an old Cadillac that had once belonged to her mother, a low wide block of a car made for long comfortable drives. 'Where would you most like to go in all of America?' she asked as we mixed cookie batter in her kitchen, stumbling over her big dog and frail Russian Blue cats, also a legacy from her mother. The dog would abruptly sit, the cats stretch out their necks and dab at his coat with their dry tongues.

Before I had time to think about the places I should see, the historical, the architectural, I heard myself say, 'Niagara Falls.' She offered me the car keys.

The Cadillac handled like a continent, huge and weighty on the road. At the lip of the waterfall the water was smooth and green, with the hardness of glass. You could almost imagine gliding over the edge. And people do; well-prepared people die at times, and the most crudely protected survive. There's a photograph of a survivor in the museum on the American side of the falls – a young schoolteacher standing in front of her barrel with a cat perched on her shoulder. She's wearing a long plain dress, the ordinary clothing of women in 1901, and nothing in her expression suggests the outrageousness of the risk she took with her life.

Really, you can live through almost anything. You can lay your head down in some very strange places. You can float to the surface of the most terrible turbulence. You can be poisoned, and in time the poison will be rinsed away.

Marilynne Robinson's novel *Gilead* is about complicated blessings, the friendship between two old men at the end of their lives, painful and resolute fatherhood; it's a book about faith and the Church. But the most remarkable baptism in the novel is a casual splashing, an event in a dream, which fills the dreamer with hope and understanding: 'I had a dream once that Boughton and I were down at the river looking around in the shallows for something or other – when we were boys it would have been tadpoles – and my grandfather stalked out of the trees in that furious way he had, scooped his hat full of water, and threw it, so a sheet of water came sailing toward us, billowing in the air like a veil, and fell down over us. Then he put his hat back on his head and stalked off into the trees again and left us standing there in that glistening river, amazed at ourselves and shining like the apostles. I mentioned this because it seems to me transformations just that abrupt do occur in this life, and they occur unsought and unawaited, and they beggar your hopes and your deserving.'

We know that this is true. Love sometimes happens at first sight. We amaze each other and ourselves. Shipwrecked in darkness, we hear the sound of the fishing boats that will bring us home. More modestly, someone makes a gesture and we see it as a blessing, we shine with liquid happiness. There are moments like this even in the depths of illness. I waited for them during chemotherapy, and during that short period of grace before radiation.

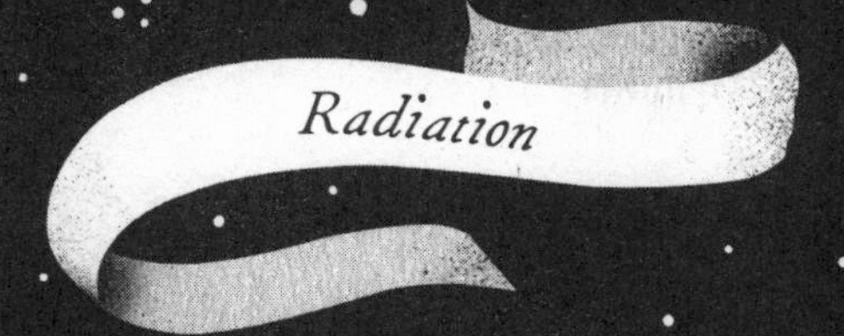
Radiation

In 1946 John Hersey was sent to Japan by *The New Yorker* with a brief to investigate the use of the atomic bomb. His essay on Hiroshima and the human consequences of military radiation, which took up a whole issue of the magazine, follows six civilians – five Japanese and one German, a Jesuit priest – from the moment of the explosion through to an afterlife of provisional survival.

The first is an office worker who is buried under furniture and books when the building she works in collapses. Her leg is crushed. She is released from the rubble and left to fend for herself, which means lying helplessly for days without food or water under a rough shelter with two other profoundly injured people. Finally she receives what passes for medical help, and a hospital bed. Someone brings her the stories of Maupassant, but she's beyond reading.

In the meantime the Jesuit priest, already weak with dysentery, has been blown from his bed where he was reading a newspaper. He escapes along with the bleeding, the dazed and the deranged, and takes refuge in a park. As he moves through the ruins of the city and its people in the days after the blast, we move with him, registering the scale of the damage. The priest is suffering from radiation sickness, which wasn't fully understood at the time. Even after the medically sanctioned radiation that was part of my cancer treatment, I was ill, and these people had had catastrophic exposure.

At one point the priest meets the office worker, who asks him to explain how God could have permitted such suffering. He says a few predictable words about sin and unworthiness, and then, Hersey tells us with great understatement, 'he went on to explain all the reasons for everything'. Sadly, there is no record of this part of the conversation. I would have liked a few handy reasons for human suffering as I sat in a waiting room alongside people with visibly painful burns, or wearing metal haloes designed to steady them during radiation. The metal is attached so firmly that blood sometimes seeps from the point where it makes contact with the bone.

My introduction to radiation procedures had come years before, when I took the daughter of a friend to hospital for radiotherapy. Horribly, unbelievably, the child had a tumour. During treatment she was alone in a room, on a bench that could be lowered or raised by remote control. She had to be positioned exactly on the bench in order to minimise damage to the tissue surrounding the tumour. Carefully measured bursts of radiation were administered by medical staff in a sealed booth, equipped with a microphone for communication. How sad it was to watch that solitary child through the window from our protected position.

After her treatments I drove her to school. I carried her from the radiation room to the car, as much for my own comfort as hers. I had held her since babyhood; my arms understood her shape and weight as if she were my own.

In nightmares our children are lost, stolen from their beds to be raised by strangers; they slip through walls that are solid to our touch. Then morning comes and we tell ourselves we were dreaming of impossible disasters. Each time I took my friend's child to the hospital, I would come home and rest on a couch, helpless in the face of this unfolding disaster, wide awake and flushed, although it was winter.

I did not know then, of course, that I would be lying under the same machine in the same hospital myself, nine years later.

Several people were involved in my radiation: the oncologist – an older Scotswoman who was so kind that she held my hand when I was first positioned on the bench – two technicians and a nurse. I saw these people every weekday for six weeks. The technicians were often young travellers, Irish or English, with the buoyancy of backpackers and plenty of traveller's tales and plans for further journeys. The oncologist, too, was looking ahead – she was close to retirement, and in her consulting room I could sense the tug of a new and less arduous life.

The hospital itself was as vast and populous as a city, and each day I made my way along a roadway of corridors to a temporary home: a TV room, a locker which was mine, a cubicle where I changed into a loose gown before going down more corridors to meet the technicians and the machine. I would lie on the bench and look up at cartoon stickers that someone had put on the equipment, perhaps to distract restless children trying to keep still during treatment. I was given two tattoos, one above the sternum, one under my arm, to help align the machine.

At first it seemed that nothing was happening. Then my skin began to burn. The weeks passed, and finally it was over. I had my tattoos clipped out at the end of the treatment and now I have small scars, like a reminder of childhood chickenpox, in their place.

This story, while true, is not so much a story as a line of defence. A wall. I'm crouching behind it, uncomfortably. During radiotherapy something invisible made its way through me, and my bones ached constantly. I was tired. I had begun to realise that cancer treatment is not really like pregnancy – you are delivered from a pregnancy, and you get back into shape. The burns on the surface of my skin healed quickly, but I was afraid that the bone pain and lassitude would be perpetual.

'This might be your lot in life,' said a worried friend, whose wife was also having cancer treatment. She was wearing his wedding ring instead of her own, her knuckles so swollen and painful that only a man's fitted her.

I began to understand that life, for some people, is a matter of unremitting endurance, something to be persisted with in order to please others. 'That is what people do. They stay alive for one another,' David Hare has Clarissa say in his screenplay of Michael Cunningham's *The Hours*. This convinces me, but it isn't enough for Richard, the sick man she's speaking to. He suicides.

If I had to nominate the single person I was staying alive for it would be my son, who came to the first radiation session with me. I couldn't see him while I lay alone on the high bench. He stood in the booth but I knew he was there, watching me, as I had watched my friend's daughter those years before. I didn't invite him, he insisted on coming. 'Nobody should have to do this by themselves,' he said. He was just fifteen.

Before going into chemotherapy, I had had a bone scan. I saw the image of my skeleton and it was somehow familiar; I could recognise my father in my basic, essential shape, and this was a comfort to me. Now a more recent scan was dappled with arthritis, as if someone had flicked ink across the shadowy grey bones, and I wasn't sure if this was a consequence of chemotherapy or radiation. All I knew was that I expected to get better quickly, and I didn't.

'Two years,' said the radiation oncologist frankly.

Two years before I could expect to feel well.

My friend Lauren tried to console me: shopping for chic pencil skirts, leaving flowers – yes, they were peonies – on my doormat, taking me to Sunday high tea at the restaurant people were talking about. Mostly I was too ill to go out at night, but she took me to see Pavarotti on his farewell tour.

He was already unwell, and although he still had almost two years to live, we knew we wouldn't have the chance to see him again. He sat on a podium behind banks of red flowers, wearing a black shirt and a scarf that broke up his bulk; he was heavy but frail, a bright doll on a stage. His voice seemed to come through him, not from him, and it was very beautiful. I sat in my little cage of arthritic pain and wondered who he might be staying alive for. His family, of course. Us, his audience, our faces wet with unexpected tears.

How to describe the emotional effects of radiation? In Berlin in the 1920s, there was a community of famous Russian exiles. The painter Chagall lived there, and Boris Pasternak, and many other writers, including the less well-known Viktor Shklovsky, who is important to me because of his book *Zoo, or Letters Not About Love*. This is a book for the suitcase, a little volume to slip down the side when you're travelling somewhere so cold that your bulky clothes threaten to split the zip. There's always room for *Zoo*. It's a series of letters to a woman, Alya, who has forbidden the impassioned writer to discuss his love for her.

So the letters are not about love.

But of course they brim with it, they leak and sweat, and because Shklovsky is such a good writer, because his letters are an attempt to win her trust, they have a bare, expressive honesty. He writes that a fellow exile weeps 'not out of sentimentality, but the way windows weep in a room heated for the first time in many weeks'. We don't write letters about weeping to people we don't love. But Shklovsky has behaved properly, strictly speaking. His emotions are kept at arm's length, and even the metaphor of the warming room is a model of restraint – tears arise impersonally due to an alteration of temperature.

Alya tries to calm him down. In a letter thanking him for a gift of flowers, she describes her room: 'The warmth, the smell, the peace and quiet, belong to me.' This is what she treasures, a solitary enclosure, free of turmoil and passion. Things aren't getting any hotter for Alya.

I thought of Shklovsky during radiation. A certain frozen stillness was part of my memory of chemotherapy: times of mad internal coldness. Radiation, on the other hand, was like an emotional thaw, a time of odd, impersonal weeping. I was like glass under condensation, a window in a room that had been empty for some time.

I worked throughout my radiation treatment. I had inherited my office from an American with a soft accent and a perfume of dark alcohol. We sent flowers when he died, but I'm not sure that any of us knew him very well. He was from Georgia – or else he was from Missouri, nobody seemed to be sure – and he seemed in some way disappointed. Perhaps the students didn't share his passion for the American novel.

When I moved into his room, the drawers of his filing cabinet opened on empty cardboard slings, each marked with the name of an American writer. I wish I had his thoughts on Melville. I do have his view, which is most beautiful at twilight, when the sky softens into violet and the river shines in the distance.

This office opens onto a busy corridor, at the end of which is my friend Michael, a philosophy professor, with a room full of unusual things. A replica of a stuffed bear, eight feet tall and snarling. Ceramic totem poles from some far region of Russia. A silver animal on an off-cut of tombstone marble. A toy acrobat carved in the likeness of Freud, from Buenos Aires. Old dark prints of the Japanese wind god on the walls. And books and leather chairs and a coffee machine.

The most lovely thing he owns is a lobster made in Kyoto before the First World War, a time when demand for traditional weapons was low and swordsmiths turned their skills to delicate and fanciful objects. Each metal segment of the lobster, every leg, is perfectly articulated, so that as you tip it about in your hands it falls open with a soft clacking sound. Michael once told me that there's only one big question in philosophy: Why do the wrong people die?

I teach a class on the novel. It's always scheduled for early evening, a tired and yet sociable time, usefully outside the pressures of our ordinary lives. Students hold chipped coffee mugs as they talk, or fall comfortably silent. Once a student brought all of Murakami's novels into class in a backpack and set them out on the table in front of him, without explanation, making an enclosure for himself. Others reached for the books – they all like Murakami – and soon the table was bare.

Apart from Murakami, they read DeLillo and David Foster Wallace and then work back to Hemingway or Faulkner. Their private, exploratory and excited reading is often American. The man from Georgia should have lived long enough to see it.

As my chemotherapy progressed, then radiation, I wrapped my bare head in various cloths and sat at tables with my students and talked about the history of the novel. Jørn Utzon's father, a shipwright, had a saying that must have sustained his son's architectural work: 'Here in the dockyard you construct and produce what you can't buy, what is not to be had, what is necessary.' Writing can be a boat, a cradle of flotation for the writer and the reader, or so I tell my students in the dockyard of my class, and some of them agree.

Nabokov advises writers to make a home in a university: 'I should still recommend, not as a writer's prison but merely as a fixed address, the much abused ivory tower . . .' The university I work in actually has a tower, although it's stone, not ivory. It's locked, and probably generally unnoticed except for the large clock on the side that faces the highway, which is useful to commuters rushing to work. The base of the tower is connected to a room that I've always liked because its ceiling is a plain white dome, like an upturned milky bowl.

Once, a student and I decided to climb the tower. It's easy to pick up the key but the entrance is hard to find. We wandered along a colonnade until workmen showed us the way. Inside the tower there was a dusty staircase, and on each landing at the lower levels we found doors that might have been false or simply locked. We tried one and it didn't move.

We climbed and climbed, stopping here and there; the height was unbelievable and the whole thing required tremendous effort. Right at the top was a final, unlocked door and a shallow ladder. Suddenly we were in an Italian space with stone arches, and a proud view of the river, the roads, the nearby hospital, and all the lesser rooftops far below. We stood on a platform of light and air. There were no safety rails across the open archways – it was dangerous and beautiful.

After we caught our breath we ran back down the staircase

without pause, down landing after landing, over a mosaic floor and out into the ordinary world.

The standard cancer mythology is a little like the view from the tower. Cancer is supposed to bring everything into proportion: small things recede, the big structures of our lives become whole and visible. This may be true of the immediate aftermath of diagnosis, but later, when life resumes, only a residue of this feeling remains. We live for our irritations, our passions, the things that loom and totter in our lives – the things we turn into the stories that keep our psyches and our communities alive. We welcome those moments when we rise above it all but you can't live up there. The best towers are locked and empty.

Around this time I came across a Paul Theroux story in *The New Yorker* about a man looking back on a personal disaster, learning from it, as we're supposed to learn from human misery: 'This whole plot – the beginning, the middle and the end – had been lived before by others, but I had to live through it myself to understand it, to know that agony can be an analgesic, that the memory of pain can itself be a painkiller. That year made the rest of my life easier.'

I hoped he was right, and that one day I would feel my experience of cancer had given me a remedy for whatever other pain might arise in my life. But I was not convinced. This is the view from above, the tower view, the view of an instructive parent, or an angel, whereas I live on the ground, which is strewn from time to time with ordinary, ineradicable human difficulty.

At one time, when my son was small, I was friendly with a man who had a gallery that sold Japanese prints. The woodblock prints I'd seen before then were recent reproductions that gave no sense of translucency. On the clean bare walls of the gallery in Perth, I saw how the old paper they were originally printed on held the light like water.

The gallery owner told me that the first copies of these prints had made their way to Europe as packing for Japanese porcelain, and they fell into the hands of painters and composers. Looking at the colours, the line, the paper itself – so perfect, so intoxicating – I had the impression that the West had been delivered, by chance, by happy accident, by distant Japan, from the grandiose clutter of its own bad art.

It isn't as simple as this, of course. The story about the packing seems to be a myth, and the Japanese printmakers were themselves working with Western ideas of perspective, but the influence of East on West was nevertheless strong. There are countless reproductions and variations of the most famous prints: Hokusai's *Great Wave off Kanagawa* turns up everywhere. The composer Claude Debussy worked with a copy of this on his wall, and chose it for the cover of one of his scores. At the time there was a mania for the Japanese aesthetic, or a French version of it, and a deep curiosity about Japan. When a painter told him that there was no Japanese word for 'nature' (which was true then), Debussy observed that 'that must prevent them from making a lot of stupid remarks'.

My gallery-owner friend wasn't given to visions of red lanterns in narrow sooty streets, shuffling, white-faced women, rooms of wood and paper and cushioned golden straw. He was drawn to the detail, the clarity and proportion of the prints, as Debussy had been, and he convinced me that I should travel to Kyoto.

It was quite a few years before I went, but eventually I decided to go one summer, when the Australian heat was at its most outrageous. Half the city drove to the coast at the end of the working day, hopped over burning footpaths to the sand, spread their towels and waded into an ocean that seemed too hot to raise a wave. Fishermen propped their rods in the sand; old people stood with folded arms, half submerged, staring out to the horizon, lost in thought. A helicopter swung overhead because there were sharks about.

The last dogs and suntanned children were herded back into the stale air of locked cars as the sky filled with pinks and orange, flaring in high rainless clouds or smearing gorgeously along the skyline. Then the sun slipped quickly under the ocean and everything was dark and huge and melting; careless, exhausted, exposed. Nobody slept, nobody was fully awake, or even fully dressed. The streets and supermarket aisles were full of salted bare skin.

In Kyoto everything had clear edges; the breath of commuters was held in surgical facemasks. I stood at my hotel window watching snow lift and tumble in invisible draughts of air; I was back in the realm of wonderment and cold. It was a generic hotel room, as unexceptional as a Holiday Inn's, but at night I kept my curtains open so I could glance out at the snow, at the strangely active darkness, and when I wasn't gazing into the snowfall, I was reading. I'd packed *The Tale of Genji*, written by Murasaki Shikibu more than a thousand years ago and often thought of as the first novel in any language.

Murasaki is said to have begun writing this tale by the light of a full moon, or so the story goes, at a temple outside Kyoto where she was nursing her grief after the loss of her husband. I read it in hundred-page chunks, with CNN playing in the background for the company of its American voices.

On my first day in Kyoto I went to a temple near the Imperial Palace Gardens, where Murasaki is said to have lived. A gravestone in the grounds is reputed to be hers. The temple garden was sombre in winter, coloured grey and the soft brown of bare trees and old timber, but there were plenty of visitors. I noticed a mother and her son, and as I drew closer the woman turned to me and said, in English, 'He wants to be a writer.' The boy beside her smiled.

'Yes,' he confirmed. He was hopeful, awkward, embarrassed by his own sincerity. I tried to ask more, but we didn't have enough words in common.

A brochure bravely claimed that the temple was 'the birthplace of literature of the world'. Did Murasaki really live here? Is she buried beneath this tombstone? What part of the body remains, after a thousand years? Her white bones? A slippery length of hair?

Edward Seidensticker, one of the translators of *The Tale of Genji*, writes: 'One can visit a spot in the northern environs of Kyoto that is described as her grave; and the marvel is that it might just possibly be.' Does it matter? We wouldn't have a passion for storytelling if we cared only for the world of facts, because storytelling is a way of adjusting the facts, of lending some and not others weight and significance, of arranging them in a time and an order that we determine for ourselves.

The facts are that present-day Kyoto is a city with Starbucks and low grey buildings and electricity poles and wires, with bus drivers who switch off the ignition at red lights to cut down on air pollution. These buses are peopled with thin old men with bristles in their ears, young men carrying babies in pouches, blond girls who've squinted into mirrors through ammonia fumes as they rub chemicals through their hair, with workers and students. Crows call overhead, droning in extended cries, or barking in short, dry-throated bursts. The smell of kerosene gathers in laneways. There's a lot of concrete.

In formal gardens, moss grows thick and deep like the bedding of lost children in some old tale. The moss is swept by men with tidy brooms. In the shogun's castle, every footfall on the walkway that links the rooms makes a sound like a flock of birds. This is the famous nightingale floor. It's not a work of art, it's a tactic to foil assassins, an alarm, a defence against sinister or unexpected movement in the building. Simple clamps and metal rods produce the noise.

This is the wonder of the place. The traveller is looking for strangeness and enchantment, for the world of clear colour on light-filled paper. Perhaps, in some temple in Kyoto, the traveller is looking for the spirit. To exist in pure strangeness or enchantment, to exist outside the body, would be terrifying, psychotic, deathly. But to see and sense these things in a busy grey city is wonderful. We need the ordinary brooms as much as we need the beds of moss.

Imagine a great black window, the kind of window a spirit might disappear through when it leaves the body. Imagine that, because of the snow, you suddenly see the way the air moves, and it doesn't move in a steady stream – as you might feel wind against your body on a hot beach – it shuffles and swerves, it's fast and energetic. You're watching the invisible, in black and white.

Then you open a book which brings you a story of a time and place you might have half imagined, in the garden of a temple in Kyoto, but because of black letters on a white page you can also regard it in detail. You're relying on thought, on skill and understanding, your own and the translator's, and other readers going back a thousand years, tracing the movement of the story.

Is *The Tale of Genji* a novel? Although it's far older, by some six centuries, than the European and English works that mark the start of the novel in the West – *Don Quixote* in Spain in the seventeenth century, *Robinson Crusoe* in England in the early eighteenth – it has the emotional scope of a novel. Genji is passionate, self-destructive; a complicated personality whose political, social and sexual world we come to understand through our concern for him. Murasaki certainly handles characterisation like a novelist. The impulse to share stories, to listen and narrate, is an ancient and profound aspect of humanity that crosses all cultures. The novel is a particular kind of story with an understanding of both the deeply hidden and socially revealed elements of human character and action, and *The Tale of Genji* shares this particularity.

But my reading of this novel cannot be precise. The text is so old, the language it's written in so profoundly different from current English. Perhaps the translator is a kind of restorer as well as a writer, a thinker and a scholar. Restorers patch, they reinforce – if necessary they use colour and line. *The Tale of Genji* is a product of devoted restoration. It took the most reliable of its translators, Royall Tyler, eight years.

Perhaps Murasaki has a similar place in his life to the place that Dante had in Beckett's. Tyler has noted: 'I was extremely lucky to be able to spend so long in intimate conversation with this great work.' When we read his translation we are listening to this conversation.

I can try to tell you the story of this immense and complicated novel in my own words, but it will be difficult, it will be like trying to track a snowfall using snow.

The Tale of Genji begins with a problem of love and politics. The emperor has fallen in love. There's nothing illicit about it: the woman has a position among his wives, consorts and intimates, but her position isn't powerful and the fact that he adores her threatens the established order. It leads to jealousy and bitterness; it could lead to political disaster.

This is something we English readers can understand – in a way, it's familiar from our Western history and traditions. We like to read about deathless love, but the social order requires something more moderate: a love that rests on faith and affection, duty and obedience. The novel is often about transforming passion into a more manageable kind of love, which is what happens in Charlotte Brontë's *Jane Eyre*. We collectively cope with extravagant intensities and intemperate lovers by turning them into stories and giving them their place on the bookshelves, where they sit quietly as the lives of saints and murderers, or as romance. Everything is safe on the shelves – in theory, at least. There vision, impulse, calculation and passion can do no harm.

But some tales of passion never quite settle down, because

they cannot be socially contained. Throughout *The Tale of Genji*, passion and determination fit into a world of manners and politics, and sometimes the fit isn't snug.

We are in Heian Japan, in what is present-day Kyoto, in a society of exquisite protocol. Women live behind the screens of blinds and curtains, occupied with poetry and stories, with writing and costume, and often with intrigue. Men enjoy these things as well, but they are able to move more freely in the world. Both men and women are constrained by distinct boundaries of class and status, established through family lineage and the adroit negotiation of marriages. Courtship takes place via the exchange of intelligent and tactical poetry, and women are glimpsed by accident or cunning. Sometimes courtship takes place by kidnapping, rape or trickery.

Sexual attraction is explained as a function of reincarnation: people who knew each other in past lives are helpless in the face of an emotion which has passed, untouched, through bodily death. Who wouldn't be? Medical treatment seems to involve a good deal of exorcism. Women who weary of court life step aside from it by becoming nuns, which involves, most visibly, cutting the hair, dressing plainly, and stepping free of the sexual complexity of the world. At times the reader senses their relief. Men, too, may settle their affairs and take an alternative, religious path. Social life in the Heian court, for all its leisure and loveliness, can require a heroic effort.

Remember the love-struck emperor? The woman he adores is not strong enough for the rancour of court politics; it makes her sick. She leaves the court and dies. In time her little son returns to his father, who makes him a commoner, placing him beyond the reach of the most intense politics: the politics of succession. This son is Genji, a brilliant and motherless child.

The emperor finds consolation in a new marriage, to Fujitsubo, who is the image of his lost love. She has the advantage of high rank, and she is less vulnerable than Genji's mother. Little Genji loves her, at first as a child and then as a man might love. When he reaches maturity he's excluded from the company of his father's women, and though he marries he still longs for Fujitsubo. His visits to his wife seem to be prompted by a desire to please his father-in-law, rather than by any great marital fondness – although, in his defence, his wife is icy and remote. The marriage is unquestionably consummated: she becomes the mother of his first son. Then she too dies.

Various sexual conquests occupy Genji, even before his wife's death, and his friends are also preoccupied with romance; they discuss their ideas about women with the earnestness of the young. In spite of all the obstacles that keep Genji from his stepmother Fujitsubo, he manages to meet her, and to her great confusion and despair she conceives and bears him a son. Genji never discovers whether his father the emperor knows of this betrayal.

Up to this point we are in the reasonably familiar romantic

territory of yearning and remorse. Then the story takes an unfamiliar turn. Genji hears of Murasaki, a child who looks like Fujitsubo. She is in fact her relative. Her mother is dead, the grandmother who's been looking after her dies, and before her father can fetch her, Genji abducts the child and installs her in an empty wing of his house, determined to be her father, her teacher and, in time, her lover. She will be entirely his.

He worries about gossip, but he doesn't seem to worry sufficiently – for the contemporary reader – about kidnapping as an act of legal and moral outrage. Nonetheless, after this unlikely beginning, Genji and Murasaki develop a genuine marriage, one of those rare conjunctions of passion and generous understanding and playfulness, all grounded in the time he spent with her when she was young. Murasaki has the confidence of a respected wife. Of course, the origin of this is objectionable from our point of view; she has never been allowed free choice. But the idea of free choice in sexual matters had no currency for many women in the Heian court.

Although Genji is a commoner he is affected by court politics, and when his father dies Genji falls out of favour and leaves Murasaki to exile himself on a remote seashore, some distance from the capital. He isn't idle, though, or indeed always alone. When he finally returns to Murasaki he must confess to a love affair with the Akashi lady, the now pregnant daughter of a provincial governor. Soon Genji has another child, a girl, to worry about, and over the next few hundred pages he steadily gathers most of the women who have been important to him, including the Akashi lady, into his household, where Murasaki holds a central position.

Late in his life, Genji makes a politically advantageous marriage to the Third Princess. Murasaki is civil about this decision, but her civility isn't effortless. The fact that the Third Princess is babyish, even foolish, helps a little. Murasaki is kind; she plays with the new wife and continues to see to all the comforts and ceremonies of Genji's life. But the additional marriage brings more than domestic tension, it is catastrophic.

The Third Princess is careless; a young noble sees her and becomes obsessed. Suddenly both are helpless: the princess because he manages to force himself upon her, the suitor because he cannot control his passion. He even steals her Chinese cat in an act of possession by proxy. Then the princess discovers she is carrying the wrong man's child, and matters come to a head when Genji reads a letter not intended for his eyes and learns of a love affair that is almost a repetition of his youthful experience with Fujitsubo. The Third Princess is ill with misery, and after her son is born she asks Genji for permission to become a nun. He allows this. The suitor, the father of the child, dies, it seems of unhappiness.

Murasaki herself is increasingly frail. With great ritual and dignity, she prepares for death. Genji finds her loss almost intolerable. He lives for a short time without dramatic incident, and then, abruptly, we are told of his own death.

This could be the end of the story, but there is a further, almost self-contained narrative which pivots on the irresistibility of resemblance, a familiar and important issue earlier on, when the emperor is drawn to Fujitsubo because she looks like his lost love, and Genji kidnaps Murasaki because of a family resemblance to Fujitsubo. Some readers may feel that by falling in love with Fujitsubo, Genji is supplanting his father in an Oedipal triangle, but there's no suggestion of fratricide in Genji's dealings with his father; and later, Murasaki is far more than a substitute for Fujitsubo. Besides, there are more interesting, non-sexual ways of looking at the situation.

Resemblance is a powerful thing. My brothers' voices, in the night, in a distant room, sound like the voice of my father. They live so far away from me, on the other side of the desert, further back along the earth's curve on the east coast of Australia. They all meet the dark three hours before I do. I may as well be in a different country.

I've always loved the places where my eldest brother has lived. I once saw in a new year in his house, alone except for my baby asleep beside me, gazing dreamily into rain and magnolias. My brother, a songwriter, works in the night. Sometimes when I stay with him I drift off to sleep to the sound of simple chord progressions. It seems to come from the foundations of our very being, his and mine. When we were children our mother played Chopin on her upright walnut piano, reprising the pieces she remembered from her girlhood lessons. She played us into sleep.

I look like my brothers. If you look like someone else, if you can slip into their clothes, it can seem that your own life is extended in theirs. You're no longer singular; perhaps you can pretend that you're no longer even finite. Sometimes, when the Sydney summer turns cool and rainy, I borrow one of my brother's jackets. I'm narrower than he is; I make a different impression on the interior of his clothes. I wear these jackets not in a spirit of impersonation, but for their warmth, their enjoyable weight and slight tobacco smell. And because in this world there's someone who looks like me. I'm not alone. Resemblance can be a fortress against the loneliness that comes with being human in a body that will one day slip into solitary death.

In *The Tale of Genji*, the pursuit of women who look like one another may be a defence against solitude, against loss and death: the dead or sequestered woman is replaced, until marriage to Murasaki stops Genji's need for substitution and consoles him for the loss of his mother and stepmother. But the final section of the novel, after Genji's death, holds no such consolation.

Two sisters are successively and intently courted by a pair of friends, Kaoru and Niou. Kaoru is not impulsive in matters of love, he's contemplative, well mannered, studious. Niou is more calculating and worldly, but each man suffers, and causes great suffering to the women they love.

Kaoru becomes the spiritual protégé of a prince, a widower who has fallen out with the court factions and has raised his daughters in seclusion at Uji. Uji is a sinister place; the prince's house is within earshot of a turbulent river, and Kaoru wonders how the prince can find peace in this location. Even the fishing is bad. After the death of their father, the two women at Uji are besieged by the young men's competitive love. The eldest dies and her sister becomes Niou's wife, but the marriage is unhappy and shadowed by Kaoru's longing for her.

In a further complication, a half-sister, Ukifune, comes to light. Each man exerts himself to captivate her, and through persuasion and trickery, both become her lover. Ukifune's unsteadiness is reflected in her name, which means 'a boat upon the waters'. Overwhelmed, she tries to escape from Kaoru and Niou; some translators believe she tries to drown herself. She's cared for by religious folk but she's lost her memory, although she does remember her longing for annihilation. When she recovers she becomes a nun, refusing to re-enter the terrible sexual turbulence of the world.

Samuel Beckett, in *The Unnamable*, the last book of his great trilogy, has a tragedy less than a paragraph long, a parody of the realist novel's preoccupation with love and anguish. It's a story about wartime lovers and suicide, complete with a bitter and compressed little coda: '. . . there's a story for you, that was to teach me the nature of emotion, what emotion can do, given favourable conditions, well well, so that's emotion, that's love . . .'

It isn't the job of literature to teach us about love. If it were, *The Tale of Genji* would contain some grim lessons, but that's not its point. This is a work that speaks of human character, of the self-destruction at the very heart of advancement in politics and love, of impulse and treachery and great remorse. This idea of fullness is put beautifully by the German critic Walter Benjamin, who wrote: 'In the midst of life's fullness, and through the representation of this fullness, the novel gives evidence of the profound perplexity of the living.' A good novel can offer a coherent account of something that is never simple, or one-dimensional – human character, and its sometimes unpredictable and unspoken motivations.

Haruki Murakami, the great Japanese novelist of our time, also has something to say about this: 'Think of it this way. Each of us is, more or less, an egg. Each of us is a unique, irreplaceable soul enclosed in a fragile shell.' An egg is a transitional thing, a promise of further life. It's exquisite as an object, but also commonplace and deeply active; eggs hatch, after all. Fictional characters, too, break free of membrane and shell; we watch them in flight in the sky of the mind. In a serious illness, when the self seems to crack a little, we might reach for a novel to remind ourselves that even when we fear being broken we are still full, still containers for the promise of growth and flight.

When I tell myself that books can save a life, I don't mean that books can postpone death. That is the job of medicine. I mean that certain books, by showing us the inner fullness of individual life, can rescue us from a limited view of ourselves and one another. *The Tale of Genji* invites us to care for a character who calculatedly involves himself in various forms of exploitative behaviour, in deception and child theft. But because we understand so much about him, from his childhood on, it becomes possible to consider him as an example of human complication rather than denounce him out of hand.

In his novel *Ravelstein*, Saul Bellow notes: 'in art you become familiar with due process. You can't simply write people off or send them to hell.' At its best the novel, as a form, resists simplistic condemnation, and it does so without paralysing the social judgement of the reader.

In the radiation waiting room, I met a woman who had learned not to condemn others. In this place the murmur of our conversation was a welcome reminder of the more ordinary complications of our lives. We talked about our work, our families, about places and people we might hold in common, and finally about the specifics of our illness. I discovered that she had been misdiagnosed when the symptoms of her cancer first appeared, and now she softly absolved the medical staff of blame for the error that would cost her life. I believe she was sincere.

I hoped that, were I ever to find myself in a similar position, I could be as generous as she was. That the valuing of complications of character, of human fallibility, would hold sway outside the act of reading, in the case of a mistake carrying such terrible, actual consequences.

Aleksandr Solzhenitsyn's *Cancer Ward* was written from his own experience of illness. After his military service in the Second World War, after his long years in a labour camp during the period of his exile in Uzbekistan, he contracted cancer.

In this novel the cruelty of Stalinist Russia has a counterpoint in the cancer ward. Exhausted medical staff irradiate themselves as well as their patients; they're beyond self-protection. We see a doctor join a queue at the market once she's finished work, waiting in line after the most gruelling day because of a rumour that a portion of sausage might be available. Characters compose themselves through conversation and flirtation, through arguments, declarations and complaints. The cancer ward is busy with words. Books are hidden under mattresses for later reading, or shared among the patients.

The ward is socially egalitarian. A pompous man who values his influence in the outer world, a man whose name ordinarily gives him access to whatever passes for luxury in the Russia of his time, feels this most acutely: 'The hard lump of his tumour – unexpected, meaningless and quite without use – had dragged him in like a fish on a hook and flung him onto this iron bed – a narrow, mean bed, with creaking springs and an apology for a mattress. Having once undressed under the stairs, said goodbye to the family and come up to the ward, you felt the door to all your past life had been slammed behind you, and the life here was so vile that it frightened you more than the actual tumour. He could no longer choose something pleasant or soothing to look at; he had to look at the eight abject beings who were now his "equals," eight sick men in faded, worn, pink and white pyjamas, patched and torn here and there and almost all the wrong size.'

As we get to know these eight men, they seem far from abject, and this man's view of them reflects more on his own character than that of his hospital companions. I've met with this attitude myself. An acquaintance, in temporary remission from cancer, tried to prepare me for radiation by telling me that the worst aspect of her own experience had been the requirement to sit in a hospital waiting room with sick people.

At one point in *Cancer Ward* a character nicknamed Yefrem is offered a book. He asks why he should read when he's about to die, and he's told to read quickly. This is the humour of the novel. Much later, Yefrem does find a reason for reading. Up until this stage in his life his reading has been largely pragmatic, work-related leaflets and a state-sanctioned account of the Party.

Then he discovers Tolstoy, and is lifted into a trance state, where he is disembodied, still: 'Yefrem just did not feel like walking about or talking. It was as if something had been stuck into him and twisted inside. Where his eyes had once been, there were now no eyes, and where his mouth had been, there was now no mouth . . . Sitting in the same position, supported by pillows, his knees pulled up to his body, the closed book on his knees, he stared at the blank white wall. Outside the day was cheerless.'

And inside? Yefrem may not be exactly cheerful, but he's sealed calmly into his body. Eyeless, mouthless, his face is like a wall; his limbs are a matter of architecture, a structure to support a book. There's no mention of his cancer.

I like this vision of the solid, dreaming reader.

The story that has transformed Yefrem is called 'What Men Live By'. The question of what men might live by occupies the cancer ward. After a little banter among the patients, Tolstoy's answer is revealed. It's love, so contrary to the rulings of the wider Russian society, to the casual selfishness of Yefrem's pre-cancer life.

Toward the end of *Cancer Ward* Solzhenitsyn has more to say about reading Tolstoy. Kostoglotov, a patient, and Elizaveta, an orderly, both have a history of imprisonment in labour camps.

A late-night conversation establishes their dreadful convict kinship, and in the course of this Elizaveta explains her fondness for French novels. Russian literature is unbearable to her; *Anna Karenina*, on the face of it a story of reckless love, infuriates her. Anna chose the path that led to her destruction and the loss of her family; Elizaveta, on the other hand, has been destroyed by the state. 'These literary tragedies are just laughable compared with the ones we live through,' she says. So she reads French novels, in French, which do not pretend to have any connection with the Russian reader. Kostoglotov asks her if reading French is 'like a drug', and she corrects him, saying it's 'a blessing'.

And what does Solzhenitsyn say about cancer? How does he reach me, in Australia, with his Russian book? He shows me something valuable that I discovered during my own medical treatment. The people who are involved in cancer – the sufferer, the doctors, the nurses, the orderlies – are often occupied less with the cancer than with each other. There are small societies of patients and medical workers in a hospital ward, and in those societies people share what they have: their love and resentment, their stories and observations. Or they sit like sturdy houses and they read.

I can't let Elizaveta have the last word on *Anna Karenina*, one of my most loved novels. It's hard to refuse the survivor of a Russian labour camp anything, even though she's only an imaginary survivor, but there are better ways of reading *Anna*

Karenina. It's not an illustration of wilful self-destruction, or a cautionary tale, unless it cautions against the easy assessment of our fellow men and women. Every character in the novel is rich in thought and impulse and vision and contradiction; every character is astounding, just as each person on this earth moves about in a day filled with the unheard music of pulse and breath, holding in their mind the shreds of the night's half-forgotten dreams, whether that person is a patient on a cancer ward, an inmate of Guantanamo, a miner in the Congo, a starving parent watching their children starve in North Korea.

If *The Tale of Genji* is the world's first novel, this sense of human largeness – where dream and memory, impulse, unforeseeable events and helpless longing are part of otherwise rational lives – has been with the form from the beginning. Virginia Woolf does this dilation of character too, but Tolstoy does it on a massive scale. If you read Woolf and Tolstoy carefully, if you agree with them about the vastness of every single one of us, you would find it hard to condemn or imprison. Tolstoy's imagination is the very opposite of that which organises labour camps.

Anna Karenina, married, with a son who can be taken from her and a social position that is vulnerable to scandal, moves by stages toward her seducer, her lover, Vronsky, and is punished terribly for her choice. When she decides, wrongly, that Vronsky is tired of her, her thoughts turn to suicide. In the end she is blind to Tolstoy's larger understanding of humanity, of the immensity of character. Vronsky is exasperated by Anna, at the same time as he is devoted to her, and preoccupied with the events and obligations of life. Furthermore he has changed; the Vronsky who cherishes the vindictive and fractured Anna at the end of the novel is a larger man than the Vronsky who pursued her in her marriage.

If she understood Vronsky as Tolstoy understands him, her suspicions would dissolve. This is an obvious thing to say, yet the gulf between the reader's sense of Vronsky and Anna's sense of him is at the heart of our experience of the book, and while many novels work with this kind of blindness, the distance between character and reader is seldom so great. Anna behaves as if Vronsky is a character in a thin romance, and that is not the kind of novel Tolstoy is writing. Tolstoy writes of Vronsky as if he were a living man.

The last paragraph of *Anna Karenina* is taped above my desk as I write. Levin, a friend of Anna's brother, and the character most prone to judgement and condemnation, has come to understand himself at last. He stands before himself in all his frailty and error, and he finds something to live by in the ordinary unreasonable confusion of his life. 'I shall go on in the same way, losing my temper with Ivan the coachman, falling into angry discussions, expressing my opinions tactlessly; there will still be the same wall between the holy of holies my soul and other people, even my wife; I shall still go on scolding her for my own terror, and being remorseful for it; I shall still be as unable to understand with my reason why I pray, and I shall still go on praying; but my life now, my whole life apart from anything that can happen to me, every minute of it is no more meaningless, as it was before, but it has the positive meaning of goodness, which I have the power to put into it.'

Those of us without coachmen, without wives or husbands will still, if we're honest, recognise something of ourselves in this. Although the power of active goodness, on its own, might seem like a childishly simple remedy to the problem of coping in this world, it's worth a try, and at least Tolstoy never underestimates the nature of the problem.

I often carry tea to my classes at the university. I sit at a wide table with my hands wrapped around the curve of china and in the small silences, the hesitations in discussion, I watch my students and think about the vastness of every one of them, about the forces of impulse and hope, of memory and understanding, that lie behind each face, and I find this comforting as I sip my tea. I find it a source of wonder and happiness.

Empathy, the way that we can place ourselves, imaginatively, in the position of another person, is at the heart of what we do as readers, as people striving for a generous understanding of one another. The failure of the party official to join the community of sick men in *Cancer Ward* is a failure of empathy, as well as a misunderstanding of the seriousness of his own illness. Barack Obama, in his memoir *The Audacity of Hope*, identifies empathy as central to his ethical motivation: 'It is at the heart of my moral code, and it is how I understand the Golden Rule – not simply as a call to sympathy or charity, but as something more demanding, a call to stand in someone else's shoes and see through their eyes.' This isn't always desirable, or possible for him to achieve. He has no sense of empathy for the men who destroyed the World Trade Center. Empathy is politically complicated.

The Australian novelist Alex Miller addresses the limits of empathy in *Landscape of Farewell*, a novel which concerns an historical event of bloody resistance. Max Otto, a German who has an uneasy relationship with his country's military past, is writing a story that his Aboriginal friend, Dougald, has given him. This story is about the killing of a white missionary by the warrior Gnapun, who possesses the ability to foresee the fates of others. In fact he can wholly enter the consciousness of other people, which he does with the missionary the night before the killing.

Gnapun lives through the dying man's agony. He understands what it means for him, a man with a loved wife, sons, and a view of passing clouds, to lose his life. He experiences this man's death as if it were his own, and yet after the vision he kills him regardless. Even empathy to the point of absolute identification will not save the missionary: a useful thing to bear in mind when we consider the functions of reading, let alone politics.

Here is a story of two readers – one Japanese, one German – powerful men with a clear sense of what it means to read. A long time ago, the Japanese emperor Saga, one of the early Heian rulers, made a copy of a Buddhist text in order to save his people from illness. Through the act of transcribing, he performed a full-bodied reading, one that took place in the wrist, the fingers and the spine, as well as the eyes. An obedient reading of an important sutra; reading as an act of ritual and sanctity, of altruism, of personal and ceremonial involvement with a text and with the suffering of others. Apparently it worked, because everyone recovered. The place where the emperor's palace stood is now the site of the Daikakuji temple, elegant, open, with walkways painted or lacquered in imperial vermilion, a colour so sweet it ought to have a taste.

By contrast, Timothy W. Ryback, in *Hitler's Private Library*, describes Adolf Hitler's reading method: 'he compares the process of reading to that of collecting "stones" to fill a "mosaic" of preconceived notions. He studies the table of contents or even the index of a book, then gleans select chapters for "usable" information. On occasion, he reads the conclusion first, to determine what to look for in advance.' Hitler, as a reader, is a predator. The book is cut up like butchered meat, and indeed Frederick the Great, whom Hitler admired, claimed to 'devour' books – a turn of phrase, and a translated one at that, but one with uncomfortable connotations.

Emperor Saga read as a saviour, Adolf Hitler as a slaughterer. The rest of us probably read as we hope to travel, flying away, losing our bearings just enough to be shown some strangeness, some wonder. Knowing we might not be comfortable for the whole journey but that we'll have something to talk about when we touch down.

It was snowing when I stood in a bamboo forest outside Kyoto, my hands around a mighty stalk. Within the stalk was a steady core of water lifting up into the sky, where birds were making their high and patient way beneath the clouds. People once believed that the crane lives for a thousand years; it doesn't matter that this isn't true. The lifespan of a Japanese crane stretches between the first novel and our times. It's a long flight from Murasaki Shikibu to me. Anything can happen in the sky.

Reconstruction

The dressing room of the pool where I do laps has a large mirror, positioned for unavoidable self-confrontation. I'm on better terms with the swimming pool itself, where I don't have to see my reflection. The lanes are separated on the surface by plastic markers. Underneath is the thick black line that absorbs you as you swim, lap after lap, in the simplified world of flotation and light muscular force, in the pleasure of the slide of water over extending skin.

Trees line the fence at the far end of the pool; there is a sense, at least half the time, of swimming toward a forest. If I'm first in on a still morning, when the image of the sky appears in the water, I have the impression that I'm sliding into clouds. The pool has seen a lot of traffic from competitive as well as recreational swimmers, and everything outside the water is shabby, except for the mirror in the dressing room. The walkways are finely cracked, the concrete is mottled, but the mirror is flawless.

In that mirror my eyes are circled in red: the impression, like spectacles, left by my goggles. I wear a black one-piece bathing suit. The set of my shoulders is like my father's, and my basic shape is the same as the women among his Scandinavian ancestors. I have a photo of his cousin Marianna sitting on a flight of steps with bowls of blueberries at her feet, the harvest from an exceptional season, and if you cover her face it could be me on those stairs.

After my cancer surgery but before the reconstruction surgery, I could stand directly in front of the swimming-pool mirror and I still looked like me. The angle, and the blackness of my bathing suit, absorbed the strangeness of my silhouette. But if I moved, it all changed. I was suddenly not myself, and it mattered. It mattered when I tried on clothes as well. I'm told that in 1697 my father's ancestor, Elias Wolker, was the wardrobe master of Charles Gustav, the Swedish king, and if there's a gene for taking pleasure in clothing, it's found its way down to me.

Think of a dressmaker's dummy, a torso on a steel pole, with or without a metal mesh skirt. An adjustable torso, so that clothing can be fitted to a replica of an individual woman's shape. Now imagine a toile, a garment made of some commonplace cloth – calico, muslin – to test the fit on the wearer. Adjustments are made to the toile, which is then picked apart and used as the basis for cutting the final piece.

Standing face on in the mirror at the swimming pool, I thought of myself as a dressmaker's dummy. Skin, musculature and bone were covered, and also disguised. I might almost have been moulded from something other than flesh. Something without component parts that could go wrong and require surgery.

My cosmetic surgeon also saw the human body as a toile – as material to be draped, adjusted, stitched and restitched, worked on until the fit is perfect. 'It's just like dressmaking,' he said when describing the procedure that would restore my shape, and although we were meeting for the first time, I knew we understood each other.

When the material being sewn is flesh, the toile itself becomes the final garment, as the healing process smooths out all surgical distortions: the edges mend together, the swellings subside. The body is both a costume, altered with skilled stitching, and solid form, the foundation for future clothing. Skin makes exquisite cloth, dense and heavy, and the seams become fine white scars.

The British novelist Linda Grant has written a book called *The Thoughtful Dresser*, in defence of the way women like me feel about the clothes they enjoy, and the way that even the most functional items – the jeans that are worn to hospital, for example – can be enjoyable. For some of us, clothes are more than just a second skin.

Tolstoy understood this. In *Anna Karenina*, Kitty, making an entrance to a ballroom, feels exactly right in her costume. She feels 'as though she had been born in that tulle and lace'. Her shoes 'gladdened her feet'. Fashionable clothes are supposed to gladden us – this is the lure and reward of pleasurable shopping – but feeling so attached to a costume that you might have been born in it takes this to extremes. At the same time, it's a recognisable moment.

Later, Kitty sees Anna Karenina's dark, sophisticated velvet gown and understands the force of understated dressing. We understand, too, the difference between Kitty's lilac ball gown, with its rosettes and swags of fabric, and the dress that the older, more socially poised Anna has chosen. Anna's gown is not plain, but it draws attention to Anna rather than to itself, and Anna is dazzling. Tolstoy tells us about the effect of a good dress from the perspective of the wearer – Kitty couldn't be more bonded to her outfit – and from the perspective of the viewer: Anna's extraordinary gown makes her beauty, not the garment, noticeable.

At its most affirmative, our choice of clothing is not frivolous, Grant argues, but intensely joyful: 'the right coat, the right dress, the right hat is like a sneeze or an orgasm, there's no mistaking what has happened'. This moment of joy has larger implications. Clothes, says Grant, may be all that an immigrant has to assert themselves in a foreign place, and adjusting clothing to suit themselves is a method of self-assertion for those making their way in the wide world – and for those who are incarcerated. Grant describes a comtesse imprisoned in the Ravensbrück concentration camp because she saved the lives of Allied airmen. Her shapeless uniform was deftly altered, inside the camp, by a fellow prisoner who had worked for Schiaparelli – dressmaking as an act of political resistance.

Like the music we listen to, like those books we keep on our shelves for many years, our clothes are defining, to ourselves and to others. When your clothes are right, says Linda Grant, 'you look like yourself and not an imposter'. We are Kitty, in lilac and rosettes, or we are Anna, in sombre and magnificent velvet. Or a woman in jeans and a cotton shirt standing before an open carry-bag, knowing that a hospital bed is waiting for her but feeling struck by the irrational sense that there's a difference, in these circumstances, between one piece of nightwear and another. That fine white lawn nightdress is going to do more than cheer her after surgery, it is going to remind her that she is herself, through the whole transition into recovery. This choice about what to wear in hospital is fundamental; it must be made even before a book is selected.

When he was a young man, Samuel Beckett put up with painful feet so that he could wear the same type of shoes as James Joyce. It was important for him to be clear about the kind of man he was, right down to his toes. Facing the mirror in the right clothes, I can say, Yes, that's me. Or waking in darkness in a hospital bed, curling more closely into the only comfortable sleeping position that a surgical drain and the tube of a saline drip will allow, I experience the lawn nightdress that lies between my skin and the hospital sheets as a slight defence against impersonality. I bought this nightdress in Napoleon Street with my friend Lauren. Or rather, we both recognised it – buying it was a matter of administration. Almost like my breath, almost like my skin, for the time that I lie here this nightdress makes me more truly myself.

Or one of my selves, because we switch between a repertoire of identities when we change clothes, as Jonathan Franzen shows in his novel *The Corrections*. 'When she put on a white blouse, an antique gray suit, red lipstick, and a black pillbox hat with a little black veil, she recognised herself. When she put on a sleeveless white T-shirt and boy's jeans and tied her hair back so tightly that her head ached, she recognised herself. When she put on silver jewellery, turquoise eye shadow, corpse-lip nail polish, a searing pink jumper, and orange sneakers, she recognised herself as a living person and was breathless with the happiness of living.'

The arresting point, for me, in this passage is the word 'living' – it points to the vitality of costume that some people experience. Couture might value pallor and thinness, on the runway or in photographs, but joyful dressing is the opposite of terminal illness. Linda Grant writes about keeping up with seasonal changes in ordinary fashion, as opposed to *haute couture*, as 'the means by which you situated yourself in the present tense' – by definition, alive.

My post-surgical shape meant that I was compromised in the wearing of clothes. I had a prosthesis, but to me it was a terrible thing: a shark fin of pink plastic, like an old doll. It made my ribs ache, and was painful resting against my irradiated chest. When my cosmetic surgeon told me that the procedure which would restore my breasts was, from his point of view, like dress-making, he also told me that the reconstruction wasn't about how I might look without my clothes on – the popular, even salacious idea of implant surgery – it was about being comfortable *in* my clothes.

My cancer surgeon had given me the name of the cosmetic surgeon during our first appointment, when I was still feeling a strange stunned alertness, as if everything were taking place in slow motion, under halogen lights. Lauren was sitting close beside me; I sensed her firm cool steadiness, which was a great feat of acting on her part. She felt much the same as I did.

The cancer surgeon had a diagram showing a cross-section of the chest wall, including the ribs, which looked distractingly culinary. I couldn't help thinking of a display case in a butcher's shop. On this diagram, he drew the shape of my cancer. I had to decide whether to just have the cancer removed, in which case surgery could proceed immediately, or have simultaneous reconstruction, which would mean a delay so that the schedules of each surgeon could coincide. I was afraid of any delay, and when I finally met the cosmetic surgeon, over a year later, my skin bore the marks left by radiation burns.

'We have to design a body for the rest of your life,' he said, as if he were an architect or a couturier, as if we were discussing a house or a classic suit, not a body. At the time I was taken by the phrase 'the rest of your life'. I was constantly frightened of the cancer recurring and I hadn't allowed myself to imagine that I would live long. The surgeon's words were a ripcord: the parachute of survival opened sweetly above me.

My cancer surgery had been confined to one breast. The cosmetic surgeon explained that, for the best results, he should operate on both, removing all tissue from the unaffected breast. This tissue, which was healthy at the time, was also vulnerable to future cancer recurrences – the idea of losing it was a great relief. The surgeon would also remove muscle from my back and use it to support new silicon breasts.

He gave me a booklet he'd written on the procedure, which included comments from his patients, and the phone number of someone he thought was a little like me, who'd just been through the whole surgical process. The booklet quoted one woman as saying that reconstruction helped her to forget she'd had cancer.

When I was having chemotherapy, another novelist who had contracted breast cancer the previous year emailed a few words of comfort to me. 'Soon this will just be a scar and a memory,' she wrote. I hoped she was right; at present the evidence of cancer confronted me in the mirror every day.

The initial surgery for reconstruction would take six hours, to be followed by several more operations. Recovery would be difficult after such major physical intervention. I could expect a feeling of tightness around the chest, where the muscle would be stretched into a new position; my shoulder joints might stiffen. Some women, I knew, were unhappy with the results, and sometimes for surprising reasons. The woman my cosmetic surgeon put me in touch with told me sternly, 'Unfortunately he cannot give us breasts that are suitable for women of our age.'

'Oh, how terrible,' I said falsely. She had overestimated me. I was fine with unsuitable breasts. Any breasts at all, in fact. Breasts are personally and culturally important. 'We are born reading,' writes the art critic William S. Wilson. 'The infant reads the breast. You cannot read but of the breast. And probably can't go to the movies, or look at a painting either.' Of course you can, but you might find yourself, from time to time, standing to one side of the general audience. J.M. Coetzee, in his novel *Elizabeth Costello,* writes that 'there is nothing more humanly beautiful than a woman's breasts' – and it seems to be a popular view. You might feel deeply alone, after breast cancer surgery, if almost everywhere you see images of perfectly matching breasts.

Without reconstruction surgery, I could never have simply had a scar and a memory of cancer treatment. I was conspicuously unbalanced; I crept about in loose clothes, or I wore the prosthesis that I found so uncomfortable. I had become a little like a transsexual, a person who feels themselves to be in the wrong body.

I once spent a few hours with someone like that. A woman who had the difficult job of preparing me for publicity photographs when *The Wing of Night* was published. At that time chemotherapy had made me deathly pale, strange-looking; I might have spooked a potential reader. She painted me in tiny brushstrokes, mixing makeup colours on the inside of her arm, wetting her brushes in the plastic lid of her bottled water, or dusting pigment from dry brushes over my skin. She was a fine painter and she made something like art of my face, something that looked extreme in the mirror but interesting to the camera and, I hoped, to whoever might pick up my book from the table of new releases and turn it over to see what the author looked like.

While she worked we talked. She had lost both parents, her mother to illness. As for her father, she told me, she was not the kind of son he had expected. And then I understood.

In the end it was Richard, the youngest of my older brothers, who convinced me to go ahead with the reconstruction. I was weighing up my options over lunch with him in Brisbane. As a child, I'd badly wanted a sister, for feminine affinity, but in conversations about breast cancer both my brothers were as thoughtful and wise as any of the women who were close to me, although nothing had prepared them for their role as counsellors.

In general I had underestimated the men around me. Male colleagues, even an elderly priest who works in Philosophy, who might have been expected to be embarrassed by such a feminine illness, sought me out. And they also found precisely the right words of comfort when our paths crossed in the tea-room or the corridor. So many lives have been shadowed by cancer. So much heart can be given in a few passing words.

Richard listened to my description of the procedure, the intrusiveness of the surgery, the implanted silicone gel, and asked, 'If you could do it in a blink, would you do it?'

'Yes,' I said.

'Then it's just a matter of time and pain.'

On the night before I went into hospital I was on the telephone to Richard, desperate and frightened and trying to find something safe to talk about.

'Do you remember Maiden?' I asked.

Of course he did. Maiden was our father's horse; she had come to the farm when he was eighteen, and when I was a child she seemed part of him, like his shaving brush. My father's parents weren't wealthy, and Maiden was a working horse, my father a hard-working boy, like a lot of children on farms at that time. She grazed on the riverbank, old and not especially friendly. I can still smell her, still see the blaze on her face, the swing of her neck when she lifted her head to look at me as I sat up high on a white-painted fence. She'd bite me if she could be bothered.

Richard and I talked about horses for a while. I had my hospital bag packed: my white pressure stockings, my lawn nightdress, ballet flats for slippers, books. I knew the surgery was going to be tough but I was more or less prepared, and this conversation with Richard was part of my preparation. I was holding the thread, the accent of my family, in my mind as I made my way forward; I could pass the time talking about horses. And then, suddenly, I couldn't do it any more. I broke and cried.

Richard swiftly assured me I'd survive the surgery, and that when I finally died of old age I'd go to heaven and Maiden would be waiting for me there. He'd obviously forgotten how mean that horse could be.

'I am the poet of breasts,' said my cosmetic surgeon grandly, and we laughed at one another. He was marking up the areas on my body that he planned to work with. He used a thick blue pen and he drew freehand what seemed to be leaves across my back and lily pads on my chest. A Balinese scene. Then I was wheeled to the pre-operative waiting room, to meet the anaesthetist.

As I lay on the gurney I watched the lights rushing past above. In the operating theatre itself the overhead light was big and opalescent, like the inside of an abalone shell. The surgeon's equipment was tucked away in a mound of dark cloth. Sharp instruments would be put to work on me; I couldn't imagine what they looked like.

The surgeon had explained that when I was unconscious, I was a problem he had to solve, like a mathematical conundrum. This way of thinking made it possible to make incisions in my living body. It was a comfort to hear this. Mathematical problems are straightforward; they get solved, or not. The surgeon likes Australian rock-and-roll, and when he operates he often listens to my eldest brother's music. I first heard these songs in recording studios in Sydney, and I remember the clean sound of the master tape, before the slight muddying that takes place with the transfer to vinyl. Everything was clearer, fresher, in the studio, and now I tried to be comforted by the idea that, twenty-five years later, this would be the music that washed over my unconscious body.

I woke from the surgery wrapped in white gauze, like the bodice of an adventurous dress. It covered my back and chest. I felt great, until the anaesthetic wore off. Then I wasn't so great.

I looked a little green, the surgeon said on his rounds

the following day. Green meant physiological outrage, convulsive misery. A blurring of thought and vision, which slowly cleared.

I was in hospital for five days that time. At night I could hear the nurses talking. Not their actual words, just a trickle of sound. Once I heard the drone and crackle of a baby crying from a place of deep, unreachable misery. The scrape of a chair, footsteps, the hushing of infantile fear. An older child called out for its mother. But I knew there were no babies, no children, on the ward. I was listening to the sounds of adult pain. I wasn't the only person suffering there.

All the immediately post-surgical nights were bad; it seemed they would never end. I had pillows under my knees, and high walls of pillows on which to extend my arms. I had a fringe of surgical drains running below the tight gauze dressings on my chest. I had to learn to sleep like this. Enthroned, speckled with bruises from Heparin injections to prevent clotting. In the mornings, nurses with needles full of this drug pinched and jabbed me. One laughed and traced a line between the bruises with her fingertip; she told me it was the Southern Cross. The Australian sky on my skin. Soon I'd have a galaxy.

My mother arrived after that first round of surgery, her fifth flight across the country since my diagnosis. She would come into the hospital after breakfast with books and a newspaper, sit in a chair at the end of my bed and read, get up to make us tea. This was always our pattern, in beach-houses and hotels and now in hospital. We read and talked. The medical narrative was taken up: what the surgeon said, what the nurses advised, what the next round of surgery might entail. I was to have four operations over a period of eight months, but the first was the most difficult, and there were times in the hospital when I wondered if I'd made the right decision.

While Richard had helped me to decide on reconstruction surgery, I'd also partly talked myself into it with the aid of Lee Miller, an American model, photographer and, later, war correspondent, who in 1930 produced two photographs of a table setting: a placemat, cutlery and a plain white plate. On the plate there sits, as a kind of meal, a medically severed breast with leathery dead skin and a glossy, jellied interior. Pictures of breasts are not supposed to look like this. Lee Miller is reminding us, quite harshly, of the diseases of the breast, and the fact that breasts are there, in the first place, to provide nourishment.

There are plenty of shots of Lee Miller's own breasts, some taken by the surrealist Man Ray. In one she's standing behind a window, the top of her gown pulled down over her hips. Her breasts are small and lovely. I propped this photo on my bookshelf to give me heart. After all, Miller knew breasts inside and out. In the first part of her life she was fearless. Then, as a war correspondent, she was one of the first to enter Dachau after the liberation and it broke her. 'I got in over my head,' she said. 'I could never get the stench of Dachau out of my nostrils.'

We cannot entirely recover from some experiences. We live through common terrors like cancer, or the horror of large-scale human destruction, and salvage what we can of our lives.

Poe has a crisp little story called 'The Man that Was Used Up'. The narrator, a nervous, bad-tempered society gossip, has his curiosity piqued by a handsome soldier, brevet Brigadier-General John A.B.C. Smith, a veteran of the Indian Wars – the battles with Native Americans. At the time Poe wrote this story there was a great deal of anxiety among settler Americans about the Seminole Wars – a brutal campaign of treachery and displacement.

Brutality is projected onto the Native Americans in this story. Smith has a resonant voice, lustrous hair, legs to inspire a sculptor. He's gorgeous, he's interesting, he talks knowledgeably about mechanical progress: 'we are a wonderful people, and live in a wonderful age. Parachutes and railroads – man-traps and spring-guns!' Poe has noticed, or sensed, the interdependencies of technological and military advancement. His character Smith is almost as bad as the Italian futurist Filippo Marinetti, who wrote that 'war is beautiful because it enriches a flowering meadow with the fiery orchids of machine guns'. Reading Poe's story in our time, knowing what we do about the carnage of warfare, Smith's 'wonderful age' is even more grimly ironic than it might have seemed to Poe's first readers.

There's some mystery about Brigadier-General Smith; he's mentioned in church, in the theatre, at the card table, with a knowingness that suggests a hidden story. The same phrases for courage are used again and again: Smith has 'prodigies of valor', but there's more to him than this, and the narrator visits him at his home to discover what it might be. He's surprised to find a mass of clothing on the floor of the bedchamber and he kicks it out of his way, provoking a bitter complaint. Smith, the perfect man, is essentially no more than a torso, a bundle on the boards.

Our narrator watches, stunned, as a slave reassembles Smith, fitting firstly a cork leg, then an arm, followed by a chest, shoulder padding, a wig and dental prostheses, naming the manufacturer of each item like any discerning and satisfied shopper. Smith is truly unpleasant to the slave, and perhaps there is some deliberate quality in this, since the Seminole were known to harbour and protect escaped slaves. The 'Indians' have scalped Smith, knocked out his teeth and cut off his limbs. But with the help of American ingenuity he is made perfect, and Poe finishes the story a little too neatly: the soldier is 'the man that was used up'.

It's supposed to be funny but Poe's humour doesn't always travel well. Like so much of his work, this story addresses fear of disintegration, and curiosity about other people's bodies.

The Indian Wars were topical in Poe's time, and slaves were a domestic commonplace when Poe was a child in Richmond, Virginia. But for the contemporary reader with a larger understanding of colonial dispossession and slavery, the story touches on a very real problem.

Cosmetic surgery has a bad name. The world is full of poverty and atrocity, people-trafficking and statelessness, and instead of making it a priority to remedy these things, our culture concerns itself deeply, obsessively, with the faces and bodies of celebrities. In Poe's story a preacher tells his congregation that 'man that is born of a woman hath but a short time to live; he cometh up and is cut down like a flower': a reminder, from the traditional order of the Burial of the Dead, of the futility of the soldier's hard-won perfection. But where do you draw the line between the vanity and exhibitionism of cosmetic surgery in the celebrity culture and the transformation that allows a cancer patient to feel at ease with their body? Cancer patients are at the irreproachable end of the spectrum of surgical enhancement, but I wouldn't be quick to sit in judgement on anyone's decision to have cosmetic surgery. I'd just like the mass media to make human rights more interesting than cleavages.

Donald Ritchie, in *A Tractate on Japanese Aesthetics*, describes a distinctly Japanese attitude to ageing and mortality: 'Many people everywhere spend their whole lives trying to escape the thought that one day they and all of theirs will be no more.

Only a few poets look at the fact, and only the Japanese, I believe, celebrate it.

'This attitude (the opposite of going to the beauty parlour) also gives pleasure – the pleasure of discovering a corroboration of the great and natural law of change in one's own personal face. This attitude extends to the outside world and seeks out a disassociated and satisfied melancholy. Cherry blossoms are to be preferred not when they are at their fullest but afterward, when the air is thick with their falling petals and with the unavoidable reminder that they too have had their day and must rightly perish.' This acceptance of change and decline is unthinkable in Western culture, although it has to be said that there is no shortage of beauty products in contemporary Japan.

The surgeon who performed my reconstruction spends part of his time in Africa repairing cleft palates, and part in Western Australia fixing up people like me. He's a long way away from *Nip/Tuck*, the TV show that parodies the glamour and turmoil of the life of a plastic surgeon. In his waiting room I met a woman who was over eighty; like me, she had been through cancer surgery. She was wearing jeans and a chambray shirt, and she looked as if she was on good terms with herself. As if she said to herself, Yes, this is me, when she faced her mirror with her new breasts. She was seeing our surgeon for a check-up.

There was a question I had to ask her. 'Are they hard?' I was curious about the density of silicone implants.

'Feel,' she said.

I pressed my fingertips to her breast. There was an initial resistance, then the softness of gel. She felt fine.

She didn't say much about her experience of cancer. It might have become no more than a scar and a memory. Perhaps she had managed to walk away from the cancer narrative.

Yasujiro Ozu's film *Tokyo Story*, set in post-war Japan, is about an elderly couple whose modest expectations of their children – hospitality, civility, the simple expenditure of time together – are disappointed. This is most acute after the death of the mother, when one son smokes slyly in the room where her body lies, and a daughter, a beautician, graspingly asks for her mother's kimono and sash. The most sympathetic character, apart from the old couple themselves, is Noriko, the widow of another son. The old man urges her to forget about his dead son, who in any case was an alcoholic and not much of a husband. He urges her to be happy. 'I'll be happy if you forget him,' he says to her. But Noriko is locked into a state of sad and indefinite expectation: 'Day passes and night comes and nothing changes,' she tells her kind father-in-law. 'My heart seems to be waiting for something.' The old man gives Noriko her mother-in-law's watch, a physical reminder of passing time.

Unfilial children appear in the stories of many cultures. What I find most touching about *Tokyo Story* is an element that is particularly Japanese. Barefoot indoors, people sit by settling back on their heels. The soles of the feet, exposed as they sit or walk, are long and beautiful. This tender nakedness is surprising to the Western viewer.

Junichuro Tanizaki, in his essay *In Praise of Shadows*, writes that 'Japanese ghosts have traditionally had no feet; Western ghosts have feet, but are transparent.' Feet are not only the emblem of departure, of the capacity to move away from grief and empty expectation, they are also, in Japan, the difference between a person and a ghost.

For me, an evening walk is a necessary part of the day. It's lightly sociable, as people nod and smile at one another on the footpath above the ocean at Cottesloe beach. A fast walk, like a fast swim, can make you feel euphoric, intensely alive – made possible by the delicate, flexible, largely unnoticed structures of the feet, which carry us along, carry us away from helplessness and stasis, into our future lives.

After my first reconstruction operation, I went to a wedding in the country. All my surgical dressings were perfectly hidden; I was beginning to get a sense of how comfortable I'd be in my clothes. The bride was one of my son's cousins, from his father's side of the family. She wasn't wearing a white wedding dress, but something pleated and emerald-coloured – vivid and unforgettable. Which was entirely appropriate, since it was just such an exceptional, eye-catching dress that brought bride and groom together in the first place.

Their grandmothers, Cherry and Pearl, had met at a country dance. In those days, girls had to travel long distances over rough, dusty roads to reach entertainment, and dresses were carefully wrapped for the journey. The dance halls had change rooms where clothing could be hung to remove the worst of the creases while the travellers splashed their faces or sipped lemonade.

Pearl, arriving late, saw a dress hanging on a clothes rail where she was about to put her own, less wonderful frock. In a way, she fell in love. Who, out in the bush, could possibly wear something so stylish, so imaginative? It was Cherry, making the most of her father's wallet and her release from convent schooling. The girls met in a cloud of organza and loose powder and became friends for life.

So were their daughters, who were the mothers of the bride and groom. Of course, the marriage wasn't inevitable. One of them could have been temperamentally unloving – some people are – or they could have simply disliked each other, or the idea of being married. They could have been gay. But perhaps they were smiled upon by the ghosts of Pearl and Cherry; in any case, they fell in love. All because of an empty dress, sadly unphotographed, hanging on a rail in a country hall.

Philip Roth's novel *The Dying Animal* is about breast cancer and unexpected love, but it's also about the significance of clothes. The narrator, David, an ageing celebrity critic who teaches at a university in New York, notices Consuela, one of the students in his class. 'Notices' is probably the wrong word, too dignified and neutral. He appraises her; she is one of many women students who, after the end of his course, when he can't be reproached for harassment, will become his sexual 'meat'.

Consuelo isn't as casually dressed as the other students, she has a blouse, a jacket, a stretch knit skirt, boots. Against all David's convictions, formed in the avid sexual climate of the sixties, consolidated by a long life of coldly passionate gratification, he falls in love with Consuela, and her clothing becomes nightmarish to him. He is in an agony of jealousy. Someone else – someone younger – might take her from him. 'I was worried about her walking around in that blouse,' he says. Her modest, slightly formal clothing is charged with erotic promise, for David and for other, younger men.

His friend George issues a cynical warning against loving Consuela. 'People think that in falling in love they make themselves whole? The Platonic union of souls? I think otherwise. I think you're whole before you begin. And then love fractures you. You're whole, and then you're cracked open. She was a foreign body introduced into your wholeness. And for a year and a half you struggled to incorporate it. But you'll never be whole until you expel it. You either get rid of it or incorporate it through self-distortion. And that's what you did and what drove you mad.'

Love is pathological, according to George. Roth himself gives us a different perspective on the pathological in this story, where cancer, not love, is the significant disease. Long after the collapse of their affair, Consuela, diagnosed with advanced breast cancer, turns to David. She's desperate, agitated, and he holds her, photographs her unmarked breasts. He's thoughtful, detached, deeply concerned. But his composure breaks when she calls him from the hospital where she's waiting for surgery. He rushes from his apartment to join her, anguished and protective, knowing that he's 'finished' – that the kind of man he has been up to this point, a man who thinks of women as his 'meat', is finally gone.

Saul Bellow, in his eponymous novel about the philosophy professor Ravelstein, comments: 'The marriage of true minds seldom occurs. Love that bears it out even to the edge of doom is not a modern project. But there was, for Ravelstein, nothing to compete with this achievement of the soul.' We'll never know exactly what Bellow means when he writes about the human soul, but the thing that he calls love may be at the centre of our experience.

Love and solitary thought can both do the work of insight and transformation. Both can bring a sense of the sweet and dangerous strangeness of other people – even, or especially, within the world of ordinary routine. There's plenty of stretch left in the subject of love, for the reader and for the novelist. And for the storyteller who deals in 'heroic optimism' – Marina Warner's term for the driving force behind fairy tales – love is often a heroic part of change.

Warner also writes about the transformations that occur in fairy tales: 'hands are cut off, found and reattached, babies' throats are slit, but they are later restored to life, a rusty lamp turns into an all-powerful talisman . . .'

My reconstruction surgery was a matter of medical expertise, fine equipment, inspiration and research, and the money to conduct these things, but it was also as strange, as unlikely, as improbably optimistic as all those other transformations.

Sarah and Lauren were the friends who helped me most during my cancer treatment, and later through reconstruction surgery. I've known both women for a long time, Lauren since the early days of my marriage, Sarah since my son was in crèche.

I met Sarah one Mother's Day. We were a sour pair, sitting on infant-sized stools while our impatient sons brought us each a paper plate of cake, which they'd been schooled to present to us by the sentimental woman at the crèche who was organising the celebrations. The boys were best friends. They'd trained themselves to eat lemons, rind and pith and all, because they'd been told to stay away from the lemon tree in the garden. This was their secret and bitter-tasting rebellion against the world of pastels and paper chains. Our sons joined a line of other children, sang a song in praise of mothers, and were then released into the garden.

Sarah, too, is a writer, and over the years we have read each other's work, passed judgement on each other's clothes, given each other advice about our sons. Both boys are only children, and we've raised them as if they're related – not exactly brothers, perhaps cousins. When I got cancer Sarah cooked for me, cared for my son, drove me to and from the hospital, welcomed my mother. Her novel *Texas* gave me a metaphor for friendships like our own.

In it she writes about Lake Argyle dam, outside the Kimberley town of Kununurra. On the floor of the dam is a station homestead, completely stocked with the large and small necessities of outback life, from machinery and saddlery to tinned baby food and toothbrushes. The valley had been flooded more quickly than anticipated, the station owners were away, and it wasn't possible to retrieve anything from the yards, the sheds, the homestead. The taps in the bathroom are still dripping, or so it's said. If you swim down you can see all this, dimly preserved, and if you hold your fingers at the mouth of a tap you can feel the slight pressure of a flow of water.

A deep friendship is like a lake containing all the small domestic memories, the accidental, the surprising, the unselfconscious moments, held as if in water. But a good friendship is never entirely still. Something fresh is continually pouring in from sources beneath the surface; a good friendship is slightly, continuously renewed.

After my final operation, when my dressings were ready to be removed, Lauren snipped away the surgical gauze with gold embroidery scissors. The dressings landed in a turquoise bowl, in a puddle of green olive oil and cotton balls. She had soaked everything in oil to loosen the tape that held the dressings in place. I should have been doing this myself but I couldn't face it. I looked away while Lauren soaked and peeled and snipped until I was bare. It was over; underneath, I was healed.

Lauren is a friend who quite simply can never be thanked enough. For driving me to hospital, for making that first appointment with the cancer surgeon when I was too stupefied to act on my own behalf. She has talked me out of mortal dread again and again. It takes some strength of character to soothe a fearful adult, to resist the contagion of fear, to soften the truth. In the early days, Lauren told me that chemotherapy is administered in a drink that tastes a little like a strawberry milkshake. She was as quick with reassurances as my brother Richard. Like my doctor, she insisted from the start that I'd make a full recovery.

People who help cancer patient have their reasons for doing so. Some have had cancer themselves. They volunteer to give massages at the supportive-therapy centre in the hospital where I had my radiation. How reassuring it is to have someone who was ill in the past slide living hands over your skin; survival seems so probable. Then there are those who volunteer as part of their mourning process, whose child, mother or best friend has died of cancer. I sometimes felt uneasy with them, as if I were a substitute for the person they had lost.

Lauren knew which surgeon would suit me best because she'd had plenty of experience with cancer. Four people close to her had had it. One, Fiona, died of pancreatic cancer, which is difficult to survive. I knew Fiona too. After her funeral Lauren showed me Fiona's sewing box, lifting out an alphabet sampler and a finely stitched, unfinished border.

Now I looked down at the small gold scissors in Lauren's hand. 'Are those Fiona's scissors?'

'No,' said Lauren. 'These scissors belong to me.'

This confirmed that her concern for me was personal, not part of some sad pattern of grief and restitution. It was as fresh as the Indian Ocean, sweeping in from Africa; as original as the sound of the master tape in the recording studio so many years ago.

Schopenhauer has a metaphor for human closeness. He writes about cold porcupines who have to snuggle up to keep warm, but if they snuggle too close they stab each other with their quills. A crowd of porcupines is constantly, uncomfortably assessing the safety of proximity.

Lauren took a big risk during my sickness. If things had gone differently, if I had had a more advanced cancer, if she had lost me, she would have been badly wounded. I saw her grieve for Fiona. I saw all her weeping. So it was good, for that reason as well, to get better, to let friendships drift and fluctuate, where once they had been so piercingly close.

It was Michael, the philosophy professor at the end of my university corridor, who told me about Schopenhauer and the porcupines. When I was sick he often invited me to his apartment in the afternoon. It's a wonderful place high above a beach, and, just like his office, is full of surprising objects. If you ever want a pigeon whistle, or the skin of a Russian wolf, or a bronze sea creature made in old Kyoto, or even the nest of a bird that has travelled through a sky you will never see, this is the place to go. Michael has plenty of American poetry and Freud; he offered good coffee or a martini.

I would sit and watch the sea. An armchair was pulled up close to the glass, from where I could look down into coral trees in which parrots squabbled and finally settled at twilight. Freighters anchored on the horizon. Or they moved too slowly to notice, until you glanced up from the coral trees and found they were in another place. Michael's cats made themselves comfortable on the windowsills, and in the late afternoon the setting sun shone through the bright red veins in their ears. I would leave my shoes at the door and settle in the chair with my feet tucked up under my skirt like a child. Michael always seemed to have the makings of a delicious meal. Crumbed Fremantle sardines. Clams and pasta. Just a small bowl, the smallest possible glass bowl, of plain ice cream.

Once I brought him a bottle of champagne with a decorative twist of wire around its neck. This wasn't the wire that secured the cork, it was positioned further down, like a necklace. 'It has no function,' I said. 'It's just beautiful.'

'Beauty is a function,' he said, and I thought about Anna Karenina in her ballgown. He was right.

As if to prove the point, he showed me a beautiful thing, a tiny red orchid. When I said it was the colour of the old cloth bindings on my collected works of Dickens, he asked, 'Does everything have to be about books?'

I thought of my parents' friend, edged into a corner by his books. What had begun, I imagine, with a sense of enchantment had ended in a kind of isolation. Too deep a fascination with any objects can take you away from the healthy shuffling movement of human society, but it can also do the reverse: it can connect us.

One afternoon after my surgery was completed, I was in my office with one of my writing students, going through her most recent work. They're usually nervous. How will it stand up, this block of pages they've put together with some intensity in a room I've never visited? A room in a share house, perhaps, with a band rehearsing in the kitchen, and a story forming on the computer screen in front of them.

My office door was open, as it usually is, so that people passing by can see through to the river. Suddenly Michael appeared. He handed me a bundle of crisp white tissue and smiled and said goodbye. The student and I unwrapped the parcel together. It was the lobster from old Kyoto, which he'd once said he would give me when I recovered.

In Beckett's story 'Dante and the Lobster', the lobster is suffering, trembling on an oilcloth table while the protagonist's aunt prepares to boil it. Belacqua has picked it up from the fishmonger earlier in the day, left it in a corridor during his Italian lesson, then handed it over to its executioner. Lobsters feel no pain, she says. Belacqua has a larger imagination: 'in the depths of the sea it had crept into the cruel pot. For hours, in the midst of its enemies, it had breathed secretly.' He slips into the lobster's shell, in a flicker of free indirect style – that point of impersonation that takes the narration directly into an alien consciousness. He speaks from the lobster's point of view. 'Take into the air my quiet breath,' the lobster thinks, or prays.

The Kyoto lobster, falling open in my hands and in the hands of my student, represents beauty and the generosity of a friend, but the lobster is also a creature that might find itself in a trap.

It signifies endurance. My metal lobster is pure exoskeleton: a shell, a carapace, a means of protection. Among its own kind, the shell is also a means of display, like a formal dress, like a costume.

What do you take with you when you slip free, as if by magic, from the lobster pot of illness?

Philip Roth's character David listens to Consuela's reaction to her diagnosis of breast cancer. 'She began telling me about how foolish all her little anxieties of a few months back now seemed, the worries about work and friends and clothes, and how this had put everything in perspective, and I thought No, nothing puts anything in perspective.' For Consuela, in the immediate aftermath of her diagnosis, everyday worries might have receded into triviality, but David, in a different situation, naturally sees things differently.

And so, four years distant from my own diagnosis, do I. When I recovered some confidence in my own health, I felt that all the minor irritations and anxieties of life – arguments, moments of carelessness, failures of judgement, bad timing, the very things I might otherwise have wished to eradicate – comprised the grain, the detail, the very story of living that I should respect. A heightened sense of the significance of narrative is what developed when I was in the trap of cancer.

Of course, narrative is not simply the details of life as it is lived; narrative is a process of observing and ordering these details, watching and shaping, and then handing the shaped thing – the story, the memoir, the novel – on to others. The Danish writer Karen Blixen understood this.

Blixen's life was made famous in the movie based on her memoir, *Out of Africa* – her marriage to Baron Bror Blixen, their farm in Kenya, the loss of the marriage, the loss of the farm, the accidental death of her lover. In later life she re-established herself in Denmark as a writer: Isak Dinesen. There's a photograph of her standing before a pair of doors in a white dress, white stockings, white buckled shoes. In her arms she has an immense bundle of white lilies. The stems almost reach her toes. The lilies have loosened a little, she's standing in a pool of white shreds and stamens. One of her buttons is undone. The light catches her wedding ring, which has the same brightness as the lilies and the linen of her dress.

In later photographs she's a different woman. Very thin. Hollow, gaunt, with black-rimmed eyes. She has a kind of chemical chic, and in fact her thinness was partly by choice. She used amphetamines, fasted constantly and adopted a stark, unsexual beauty. But her weight was also a consequence of illness: syphilis, contracted in Africa.

Blixen understood a great deal about suffering, about the lies we might tell ourselves and one another, and she also understood the way humans are drawn to the sea. She writes about shipwrecks and voyaging, about castaways whose islands are bad marriages or other kinds of exile. 'There is nothing for which you feel such a great longing as for the sea,' she writes. 'The passion of man for the sea . . . is unselfish. He cannot cultivate it; its water he cannot drink; in it he dies. Still, far from the sea you feel part of your own soul dying, disappearing, like a jellyfish thrown on dry land.' Of all her stories about seafaring or strange travel, my favourite is 'The Pearls'.

Jensine is a young Danish bride who goes to Norway for her honeymoon. She is happy to be married, she is in love, she wants to be alone with her husband in this wild and precipitous landscape. Paris, the obvious place for a honeymoon, has no appeal for her. But in Norway she discovers that her husband is intolerable – not cruel, just wholly superficial. 'Now she felt, with horror, that here she was, within a world of undreamt-of heights and depths, delivered into the hands of a person totally ignorant of the law of gravitation.' She isn't, of course, talking about the scenery.

The newlyweds climb together. Jensine takes great risks in an effort to jolt her husband into some understanding of jeopardy, of depth, but it doesn't work, he simply admires her courage. The honeymoon becomes a matter of 'strange warfare'. He doesn't even know he's in a fight. Just before they return to Denmark she accidentally breaks a strand of pearls he has given her. The necklace once belonged to his grandmother, who received a pearl for each wedding anniversary. They're a kind of abacus, a counting device for the years of marriage. They're also quite valuable.

Since there is no jeweller in the town, Jensine is directed to a local shoemaker who has the skill to repair her pearls. Two years before, he fixed the pearl necklace of an aristocratic English couple. The shoemaker is wise and austere; he had hoped to be a scholar and a poet, but his dreams came to nothing. After leaving his workshop Jensine has a conversation with another Danish traveller, a Herr Ibsen, who tells her that the shoemaker has a great many pearls. This is of course metaphoric: Ibsen is a famous playwright, he's collecting folktales and the shoemaker is one of his sources.

When Jensine recovers her necklace, her husband suggests she count the pearls – the shoemaker may be a thief. By now she considers her husband to be a fraud, and in a spirit of superiority she refuses.

Some time later, back at home, Jensine does take up her necklace and count her pearls. It has indeed been altered. Bafflingly, there is an extra pearl in the strand. Far from being robbed, she has been enriched.

She writes to the shoemaker in an effort to clear up the mystery. He replies explaining that he accidentally failed to restring all the pearls in the Englishwoman's necklace, and because he couldn't contact her to return her pearl he added it to Jensine's strand.

'The Pearls' is not a story about the value of settled marriage, the accumulation, in time, of lustre, as the title might imply. Rather it's a story about storytelling. Ibsen has told Jensine that the shoemaker has a stock of pearls, of stories. Her necklace will be passed to another bride, in a hundred years, along with a tale of marriage.

It's also a story about distance. At the end, Jensine and her husband are looking down at the street below, from quite different windows. The lesson of Schopenhauer's porcupines – a lesson of necessary human distance – comes to my mind, but this is more than a little social distance, it's a temperamental estrangement between husband and wife. Yet 'The Pearls' is not desolate; it isn't about failure, it's about our tender connection with the unborn, with unknowable future lovers who will inherit the narrative treasure of the family. The particulars of character – the stupid man, the contemptuous bride – don't matter. Only the gift of narrative matters.

Pearls grow out of grit and injury. They're smooth globes of healing from under the sea. Blixen writes that 'pearls are like poet's tales: disease turned into loveliness, at the same time transparent and opaque'. Disease turned into loveliness indeed. Not all stories form around disease, but most have a central irritant.

I got better. And something grew in me: not a cancer this time, but some increased concern with the thing I do, the telling of stories. In *The Thousand and One Nights*, Scheherezade, under sentence of death by her husband the Sultan, postpones her execution by telling him a story. But the story is not resolved at dawn, and as he cannot bear to miss out on the ending he lets her live. And so it continues with the next story – Scheherezade's stories are her salvation.

As an habitual, even occupational reader, I know that death can be a way of finishing a novel, or beginning one; it can be central to plot. But as a writer, I feel that storytelling is about staying alive. All narration holds the promise of further stories, and another dawn.

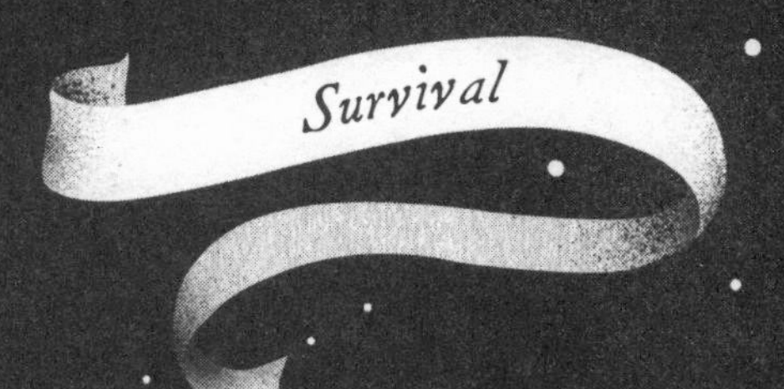
Survival

It was some three years after my diagnosis before I felt I'd come back home again, to my seat at the long white writing table in the room with sandstone walls and wooden floor. It's a kitchen table really, painted inexpertly by me and winched up to the second storey through the French doors by reluctant removalists. All that effort for such a poor piece of furniture. But its slab of whiteness is like glossy paper, faintly ridged by my brush-strokes, striated with the reassuring markings of an earlier self. It's a marker of continuity, of survival: a gathering together of the time I acquired it and the here and now. I've been dislocated for a time by cancer, and now I'm not only a different person from the woman who painted this table, I'm different from the woman I would have been had I never fallen ill.

My hands hesitate above the keyboard. During chemotherapy, and for some time afterwards while my health was being closely monitored, I had wads of cotton wool taped to the crook of my arms, and when the veins there became unusable, on the backs of my hands: little stoppers for the places where the medicine had entered my body, or where blood was taken for testing. Now that's all over and this particular evidence of my illness is gone. Later in the morning, when the dawn chill leaves the air, I'll open the French doors, and if I'm very still rainbow lorikeets will land on the trees and lever themselves along the branches using their beaks and claws, moving as if swinging from a trapeze, too lazy, for the moment, to flap their wings.

I work at this table at night as well, when I can look out and see the moon in her various phases. Sometimes it's a horizontal crescent moon, like the lower half of a wineglass, which my father calls a water moon. How calming it is to watch the moon through the branches of familiar trees, to know that a diminishment in its form will return, in time, to fullness. Here is something we can trust, for as long as the earth and moon endure.

This is what I most hoped for after I was diagnosed with cancer: calmness, this position at my table and, above all, time to raise my son. Of course I also wanted more, particularly books: all the books I looked forward to reading in the future, and the books I imagined I might write. It's all so commonplace, yet so much had to happen, over such a long time, before I could resume my early-morning place here, in my old and pleasurable routine, in a body I never expected to have.

This body governs me strictly. If I drink much alcohol I ache and burn with thirst. Too much sugar affects me as I imagine amphetamines would, causing blazing alertness and insomnia. If I sprint through my day my feet prickle with pins-and-needles, and go numb. Without my favourite clothes, laughter, motherhood, I'd feel confined indefinitely to a repressive boarding school.

I think the prickling and the numbness are after-effects of chemotherapy. The aching began during radiation, and improved, over time, but it can return. My lack of stamina is caused by loss of oestrogen. In survivors of hormone-sensitive cancers, such as breast cancer, oestrogen must be suppressed. Each night I take Tamoxifen, a drug that lowers the oestrogen level in my body and ensures that the following day will be a little slow. As one GP explained to me, it's oestrogen that gives you your bounce. So I try to move steadily through my life now, remembering what it was like to bounce.

My new body, so severe in many of its habits, also carries permanently adolescent breasts. Breast cancer has another unexpected connection with adolescence: one of the things that apparently predisposes women to this disease is being tall at around the age of fourteen. There seems to be no explanation for this, but it certainly applied to me. I was five-foot nine, in the old measure, and I grew another two inches before I turned twenty. At fourteen, too, I had a fair idea of what kind of body I'd have in adulthood. Sleeping in my genetic code were instructions for barely imaginable volumes of flesh and lengths of limb, which appeared in unpredictable spurts of growth over a few short years, before all the changes slowed. For everyone, adolescence is an exciting, frightening, often disappointing time. Nobody ends up exactly as they'd wish to be.

After my cancer surgery, and the six hours of reconstruction, the months of further operations and procedures, something like the process of adolescence happened all over again, but this time I had choice. The size of my breasts was up to me; I even picked a colour for the areolae – a bit like choosing a lipstick. And instead of the delicate, invisible, long-term interactions of hormonal biochemistry, on a certain date my name simply appeared on a surgical list. My new breasts began on that specified day and were finished on another, in the rooms of a medical tattooist whose needles created bloodied carmine nipples that healed in time to a natural paleness.

It was Lauren who took me to the appointment with the tattooist, rearranging her workload to do so. The tattooist worked in a suburb by the river that was full of old jacaranda trees. They were in flower, their masses of purple blossoms contrasting with terracotta roofs. In places they formed a canopy high above the road, and we drove away afterwards through arches of sweet colour, both of us purely happy – Lauren because she had seen me through to the end of all this, and me because of my dramatically bright and finally complete breasts. A few weeks earlier, my cancer surgeon had told me he couldn't declare unreservedly that I'd never get cancer again – there are no contracts for this sort of thing – but he believed this would be the case.

There is a small price to pay for a second set of breasts: they can never feel like a natural part of the body, they are almost completely numb. A woman I know who had reconstruction surgery sent me a card with best wishes from herself and her small plastic breasts – this is how she put it, as if they were another entity, separate from herself. And indeed, there are times when my own breasts seem to be the property of my cosmetic surgeon, especially when medical staff examining me recognise his work and name them as his.

There is another kind of estrangement that comes with the post-surgical body. Some people are confrontingly curious. Knowing I've had cancer, perhaps knowing I have reconstructed breasts, they look swiftly at my chest during conversations. The breasts have briefly cancelled the person. It's a forgivable impulse, of course, but just as understandably, I don't like it – it adds to the feeling that my new breasts don't quite belong to me.

The time I'm most thankful for the work of my cosmetic surgeon is summer, when I can walk on the beach at twilight in light clothing, through crowds of strangers in bathers and towels, past dogs and fishermen and late kite-surfers. Bodies are exposed, yet most people are tactful about where they look, are careful not to appraise one another offensively. I can wear a camisole with my rolled-up jeans, or a cotton dress with shoestring straps – I can be comfortable in the heat.

These beach walks are an exercise in happiness. On the beach in summer I can barely remember my immersion in the waves of panic that accompanied my illness. This is not a fragile euphoria, but a steady sense of happiness, and it runs deeper than relief at the fact of my survival. I see it as an evening-out of the emotional balance of my life, after having lived, for that period of the cancer, with such fear.

For the four years from 2000 to 2004, I sat at my white table writing a novel about war, imagining what it might be like to fear for your very life, to be helpless in the face of imminent physical destruction, unaware that the question of survival would soon be so close to home. When I tired of my novel I could put it, and the question of fear, aside and work on something else. But then an all too real fear came to rest in the place where my heart lay, and there was no escaping it; it seemed at the time that my heart was cupped by fear. Where once I had imagined women farewelling men in uniform, now I understood that I might be forced to part unwillingly and forever from my son. I was no longer directing a story, I was within it, and I had little control over what took place.

Warfare is such an established part of the way we think about responses to sickness that the metaphor can lose its meaning. We talk about people dying after long battles with illness; patients are encouraged to visualise their body's defences attacking a disease. But the comparison does have force and usefulness. A combatant has a more powerful role than a patient, and I tried to see myself in this way. In my cancer treatment, the larger strategies for survival were determined by professionals, and while I was not a brave soldier – I felt I had no courage – I knew how to compose myself and do as I was told. To endure. And perhaps the same is required of military personnel. When I was sick I felt like a soldier who understood, urgently, that sudden death is possible. Before my sickness I was, in relation to death, a civilian.

In *All Quiet on the Western Front*, that most graphic of war novels, a German infantryman on leave from the trenches returns home to find that his countrymen want to hear dramatic stories of military adventure. But Paul has had too much adventure; he values stillness and calm: 'Sometimes I sit with one of them in the little garden of the pub and try to get the point across that this *is* everything – just sitting in the quiet.'

When Paul and his fellow soldiers were marching to the front, they passed a school that had been destroyed by shellfire. Some hundred pristine coffins rested against what was left of the building, and Paul and his friends understood that they were looking at their own coffins. This is the lesson the ruined school teaches them – that they will die.

They are very young, just eighteen. Such a short time before, in their own classrooms, they were reading Schiller and Goethe. Now they must listen carefully, because their lives will depend on identifying the sound of particular shells. Yet on the front-line they will be deafened by the noise of bombardments, their auditory defences will be lost. There is also the constant risk of live burial as shellfire destroys dug-outs and trenches. In an earlier confrontation, a cemetery was shelled and the living were mixed appallingly with the contents of graves. Splinters from exploded coffins were used to stabilise broken limbs.

Coming home on leave to the civilians who want him to tell the kind of story he cannot frame, Paul is at first unable to speak at all. Later, he stands in his own room like a stranger, remembering the effort he had to make to buy his small library. He takes up the position of a reader: 'My hands are lying on the back of the sofa; now I make myself comfortable, tuck my legs in and sit easily, cradled in the sofa's arms. The little window is open, and shows me the familiar view of the street with the church spire looming up at the end. There are a few flowers on the table. Pens, pencils, a shell for a paperweight, the inkwell – nothing here has changed.'

Paul is describing the kind of place we readers all inhabit. Here is pleasure, the future, the youthful past. Briefly he imagines that the war will not 'devour' him; he believes that men like him will return safely home, that 'the war will sink and drown when the wave of our homecoming sweeps across it'. Then he loses confidence. The books, the pages in his hands, mean nothing to him. He is compelled to leave his room.

All Quiet on the Western Front shows a reader, a hopeful man, destroyed by terrible circumstances, but we on our sofas, with our own few flowers on the table, are not destroyed. We keep reading about the character of Paul in a book that tells a story of the failure of storytelling, at the same time as its power is being demonstrated.

Paul's silence, his detachment from the things that once gave his life its savour, are familiar to me from the time I returned to my house immediately after being diagnosed. I saw all my possessions as meaningless, or worse, as burdened with sadness, and I imagined my son looking through photographs that would, if I lost my life, be memorials, not casual records of events.

I spoke to very few people at that time. At first I planned to keep the bad news from my family, who all live so far away. I thought I could just tell Lauren, Sarah, and one or two people at the university, the people who were immediately necessary to me. I would slip away for surgery, take extended leave for chemotherapy. Safety seemed to lie in privacy; once the situation was openly acknowledged, it would become real and terrifying.

Before going in for surgery I could barely bring myself to believe the diagnosis.

But the story was uncontainable. When Lauren changed her teaching schedule to take me to my first appointment with the cancer surgeon, the colleague who replaced her was indiscreet. And although I could barely find the words to explain my situation, I also had a selfish, heartfelt need to tell my family. Later, I came to see that hiding in silence is not the same as being safe.

Many men who returned from the Western Front at the end of the war found a way back to the things that had given their lives meaning before the war; they took up their books again and lived altered but satisfying lives. Books won't prolong my own life, but they won't shorten it either, and reading beside a door that opens onto the branches of a tree is a fine way to spend some of the time that good medicine has obtained for me. Reading reminds me that we are not so singular after all, that there are crowds, whole populations, in the stack of books at the end of my table. Some of these people will trouble me, some will appear in thoughts and dreams, and they will all still be here, Malone and Anna, Genji and Paul, when my own books are out of print, when my writing table is just another chipped piece of furniture at a clearing sale.

The artefacts that remain after the end of an ordinary civilian life like mine are usually discarded, but those of soldiers acquire special significance. It's as if the keeping of mementos, the conserving of objects – badges, weapons, even boot-leather – might weigh against the profligacy of wartime destruction. The battlegrounds where men like Paul lost their lives are excavated now, and the items discovered there cleaned and exhibited. The Western Front was an appalling place in 1918; photographs show men so thickly encased in mud they look as if they've become the very substance of the battlefield. The division between flesh and earth is lost.

The fighting in coastal Papua New Guinea in the closing stages of the Second World War also took place in wet and quickly defiled terrain, and although the scale of the casualties of the two battlegrounds are not comparable, both share this horrific conjunction of flesh and dissolving earth, of men floundering on unreliable ground.

In 1943, as the Japanese campaign in Papua New Guinea collapsed into a nightmare of malaria and starvation, the mess tins of Japanese soldiers acquired a formal, ritual meaning. The Japanese Imperial Army addressed the problem of repatriating the dead by sending relatives the ashes of some fragment of the body in the soldier's tin. When even this much was impossible, families received empty tins. It was believed that these contained the spirit of a son, a brother or a husband; that they nourished people in their grief.

The soldiers themselves, holding empty mess tins in the fouled swamps and high country of New Guinea, could not conjure solid rations. They starved; some resorted to cannibalism. There are accounts of the discovery of human meat in the cooking utensils of Japanese soldiers at Sananda. This was survival in extremity, and one prisoner of war under Australian interrogation spoke of the despair of those who had eaten human flesh 'when they realised the full significance of their act'.

Cannibalism is not only a matter of survival in the worst imaginable circumstances, it's also an act of self-annihilation, the ultimate collapse of individuality, one person subsumed in another. Part of the horror of cancer is that it is a form of biological self-destruction, a disorder wherein malignancy colonises healthy tissue. The body turns upon itself, becomes a battlefield, a tract of unreliable ground where normal divisions fail.

And just as the origins of major conflicts are often indistinct, or lie in cumulative and seemingly unrelated provocations, so too are the causes of many cancers difficult to pin down. Over-consumption of alcohol, excess weight, a family history of the disease are among the other factors that can predispose you to breast cancer – although I seemed to have none of these. Sometimes destruction just comes without warning, like the fascist bombing of the civilians of Guernica in 1937.

When I was pregnant with my son, the military conflict of the Gulf War seemed to contradict everything my body was engaged in: the unconscious creation of new life. With my cancer diagnosis came the realisation that malignancy and internal biological destruction were also part of me; I suddenly contained a kind of war.

Of course, the comparison between war and cancer is hubristic – the contraction of cancer is not a national matter affecting entire populations – yet fear and negotiation, resistance and the terrible possibility of surrender are part of the experience, so that cancer can seem very much like an interior war. When I was diagnosed I made private pleas and treaties, hoping for a position at my table: here, in the quiet space of early morning, broken by the bell-like calls of parrots as they make their way to the Norfolk Island pines beside the beach.

Shortly before the eighteenth-century philosopher David Hume died, he had a conversation with his friend the philosopher and economist Adam Smith. Hume, who knew his condition was terminal, joked about gaining a little more time for himself by striking a bargain with Charon, the ferryman who carries the dead to the underworld in Greek mythology. 'I thought I might say to him, "Good Charon, I have begun correcting my works for a new edition. Allow me a little time, that I may see how the public receives the alterations." But Charon would answer, "When you have seen the effect of these, you will be for making other alterations. There will be no end of such excuses; so, honest friend, please step into the boat."'

No book, no story, can buy the kind of time we all want: to see our children grow to adulthood, our grandchildren; to linger in our lives, see where our ideas take us. Yet literature abounds with stories that defend against death, *The Thousand and one Nights* being just one of many. 'By Allah I will not slay her until I shall have heard the rest of her tale,' says the Sultan as Scheherezade's wedding night draws to a close.

In Boccaccio's *The Decameron*, written in the fourteenth century, a group of young Florentines avoid the Black Death by quarantining themselves outside the city where infection is rife, and the book details the stories they exchange. This tiny society of listeners and storytellers is like a vessel of survival – self-contained, fitting together. The listeners are also speakers waiting their turn. The characters are a little like each other's readers and writers, which means that the reader of *The Decameron* – you, me, anyone with a copy of it in their hands – has a symbolic presence inside the text, a space which has deliberately excluded death. This book is a reminder that the storyteller doesn't have a monopoly on the exercise of the imagination; it's based on the understanding that the reader is a storyteller-in-waiting.

J.M. Coetzee's *Foe* is a novel that works with a similar idea. It's in fact a novel about a novel, a variation on that most famous of survival stories, *Robinson Crusoe.* In it, Susan Barton, the vagrant widow of a castaway, imagines a writer called Foe at his shabby desk at the top of a house besieged by creditors, in an attic overrun with vermin. It's London in the seventeenth century and the character Foe is Coetzee's version of Daniel Defoe, who wrote

Robinson Crusoe. In *Foe*, Coetzee, whose work is often engaged with literary history, is both reader and writer in one.

The protagonist of his later novel *Elizabeth Costello* uses the same device. She is a novelist whose most successful book springs from James Joyce's *Ulysses*. Elizabeth explains to an interviewer that 'certain books are so prodigally inventive that there is plenty of material left over at the end, material that almost invites you to take it over and use it to build something of your own'. Perhaps something similar has happened with *Robinson Crusoe* and *Foe*.

Susan pictures the writer Foe at the helm of a decrepit ship: 'I think of you as a steersman steering the great hulk of the house through the nights and days, peering ahead for signs of storm.' The image is a sinister one. Historically a hulk was a prison anchored in the Thames, confining those convicts spared the fate of execution; it was the very opposite of the Ark. And since Defoe's *Robinson Crusoe* is an account of shipwreck and ingenious survival, the vision of Foe at the wheel carries a sense of impending catastrophe: a hulk is unseaworthy, there must be a shipwreck before the story of survival can begin. There is something comforting in this for the reader who has faced their own catastrophe.

In Defoe's novel, the solitary Robinson Crusoe discovers a footprint in the sand. Is it his, preserved from the time he came ashore after the wreck? If so, he's discovered a memento of his own salvation, a cheering marker of survival. Or is it the impression left by a stranger, a cannibal? Crusoe measures it against his own foot – it's larger, the print of a trespasser, and immediately he's shaken, trembling with fear.

All survival is ultimately provisional. The footprint of the cannibal, warning that we may be swallowed up, and the prints left by our own feet as we make our way to solid ground are equally extinguished. We are all finally engulfed. In the survival story, death is only glimpsed, at a necessary distance from the self, but real life is not so kind.

Foe begins with a landfall. Susan Barton has been set adrift in a rowboat after a mutiny on board a ship bound for England. When her hands are no longer capable of working the oars, she abandons the boat and swims to an island. Waves sweep her in to shore, where all her efforts cease. 'There I lay sprawled on the hot sand, my head filled with the orange blaze of the sun, my petticoat (which was all I had escaped with) baking dry upon me, tired, grateful, like all the saved.' The island is inhabited by Cruso, a far less adventurous and enterprising version of Defoe's Crusoe. Susan reports on what she finds: a taciturn man who builds futile terraces for a crop he doesn't have the seed to sow, and Friday, a mute slave.

Redemption comes not through industrious and fruitful toil, as is the case in *Robinson Crusoe*, but in the form of a passing ship bound for England. Having found lodgings in London, Susan seeks out a writer in order to make money from her story. This writer is named Foe, Daniel Defoe's original surname, which stands as another point of affectionate antagonism between *Robinson Crusoe* and *Foe*. Cruso has died on the voyage home and Friday is now Susan's bewildering responsibility. She herself is a thorn in the flesh of the adventure story, interrogating Foe on the need to adjust the truth so as to satisfy readers.

The island she knew was a dull, monotonous, windy place. Must she invent a tale about cannibals? Foe, according to Susan, 'knows above all how many words can be sucked from a cannibal feast, how few from a woman cowering from the wind'.

Robinson Crusoe works in part because Defoe convinces us of the landing of cannibals on Crusoe's shore. If we lose faith in these cannibals, if they seem like an expedient plot device, we may also lose a little faith in the book. Foe, novelist and creator, is taxed by Susan with almost theological questions of what makes a vital, readable and credible story, of how a life and a story might part and join, in the interests of the survival of each.

He tells Susan a fable, a moral tale from Newgate Prison. A woman who is to be hanged asks for permission to make a confession of her sins: such confessions were published as broadsheets and widely read in Defoe's time. She details thefts, infanticides, multiple acts of bigamy – her wickedness knows no end – and then proceeds to cast doubt on the truth of her own lurid story. And since she's lying to her confessor, that too is a sin that must be revealed. She isn't given the chance to do this, but it's an ingenious strategy. For as long as she talks, her execution is delayed; confession is her life raft and her buoyant wave. The impatient chaplain breaks in with a premature absolution and she is led away to the cart and the scaffold.

Foe and Susan debate the meaning of this story. For Foe it's about the need to resign ourselves to death, for Susan it's about the harsh exercise of power. For the reader it is also, of course, a survival story, of the kind Hume imagined telling Charon. No wonder Susan Barton sees Foe as the steersman of a hulk, holding a course for as long as the timbers can withstand the pressure of the swells.

Robinson Crusoe, stranded on his island, struggling against self-pity, asks himself, 'Is it better to be here or there? And then I pointed to the sea.' We like to stand on dry land within sight of the waves that have failed to close over our heads, even when we haven't fought our way clear of a wreck. Of all the reasons why we lie and walk on the sand, and swim under the eyes of the lifeguards, this might be the most atavistic: we are safely here, on solid ground, and not there, in treacherous waters.

Coetzee concludes *Foe* in a way that entirely releases the novel from realism. The final pages are recounted by a nameless storyteller who enters Foe's house, where Susan and the writer lie facing each other, dead, positioned with tenderness. Friday, too, lies dead in the same room. The manuscript of the novel *Foe* is discovered in a box on the floor. The storyteller reads a few lines written in Susan's hand.

In dreams we have the power to slide through folds of time, travel to distant places, fly. The anonymous storyteller at the very end of *Foe* has this dreamlike power to move unhindered through physical and temporal obstacles, observing an alternative story to that told by Susan, the story we have been reading, and believing, up to this point. The sex of this later storyteller is not revealed: he or she is suddenly within the world created on the first page of the novel, slipping over the side of a rowboat, just as Susan did, within sight of the island we recognise as Cruso's kingdom. But instead of swimming to the shore, this storyteller finds a way down to the seabed, where the wreck of Susan Barton's ship has lain for three hundred years.

Is this the truth of *Foe*? Was there no mutiny, no landfall? Or are questions of truth beside the point, which is to represent the power that lies with all readers, the power to imaginatively swerve away from the designated story and invent yet another for themselves, perpetually revising, like the condemned woman in Newgate Prison?

Of course, in real life it's never that simple. At the point of diagnosis, the cancer patient is forced to hear a terrifying story involving surgery, chemotherapy, radiation. When the story finishes the terror remains, paralysing the imagination, preventing the perception of any ending other than an early death. Fear must be stilled, self-confidence marshalled, until the paralysis abates, the story of imminent death passes, and more hopeful stories take its place.

Medical studies acknowledge that the worst period, emotionally, for many cancer patients is just after treatment finishes. The cold, intermittent sense of dread that I experienced following my diagnosis occurred when I was still in shock. But I was almost disabled with fear when my radiotherapy finished, because this meant there were no more remedies. It was now up to me, to the resources of my body, and I saw no reason to trust the body that had already let me down. I felt shadowed by a horror that was also a part of me. I had unnecessary tests to check for recurrence, and I came out of each one with a sense that I'd passed an examination. But my relief would be short-lived. I talked constantly about these tests, which was boring for other people and unhelpful for me. I couldn't have told a story to save my life.

In the end, I found that the things we tell our children to comfort them in the night can also console us: things *will* quite often be different in the morning.

A woman I know who went through cancer treatment months before I did told me at the time that for the rest of her life she would feel the hand of death on her shoulder. Now, five years after her diagnosis, she has set up a household in a new city. She's always in a meeting or on an aeroplane. Last time we spoke she was about to serve dinner, breaking off the conversation to toss instructions to her children, and if she gave a thought to her own mortality I'd say it was a passing one. For myself, I find that there's value in knowing that I have a *life* – beginning with the rush of oxygen into new wet lungs at birth, and ending with the final subsiding of breath and tissue. The decisions I make are just a little more considered now because I know, intimately, that my life will end.

An historian at my university who had breast cancer eight years ago died early in 2009 after a recurrence. Someone put a huge crumpled garden rose in the slot of her letterbox, which was in a busy corridor near the bathroom on my floor. Whenever I walked past the rose I was touched, sad and frightened all at once. Michael, who understood exactly how I felt, said sensibly, 'Why don't you use another bathroom?'

In time my fear receded, and I could think about this woman's voice, her smile, her fine work. At the spring 2009 graduation ceremony I watched her last students cross the stage to accept their doctorates, and her death did not seem at all like a harbinger of my own.

At the end of *Foe*, Susan and her captain are shipwrecked, drowned and still floating near the ceiling of their cabin. Deeper in the same wreck, the narrator finds Friday and prises open his mouth. Speech is of course impossible underwater, but Friday's mouth releases an intimate current, a stream of water that plays on the face of the storyteller, palpable and diffuse, like a spring. His discharge issues in place of words; his own story remains beyond interpretation.

Robinson Crusoe, the foundational English novel of survival, is, in Coetzee's hands, about far more than an enterprising individual. The 'material left over at the end', to use Elizabeth Costello's phrase, becomes another story, a story for contemporary readers. Of course this could not be done if *Robinson Crusoe* itself were not so fascinating, so alive with questions for the reader.

Beckett's *Malone Dies*, with its solitary wrecked old man, occasionally taking an 'inventory' of his possessions, amounting to little more than a notebook, a pencil, a stick and a view from a window, is a parody of *Robinson Crusoe*.

I have a great affection for novels like *Foe*, which hover above existing works of literature like a magnifying lens, producing a particular kind of clarity. Not everyone agrees. Julian Barnes, in *Flaubert's Parrot*, has his protagonist list novels that should be prohibited. Castaway novels involving cannibalism come first – they're too easy, and not much fun, apparently – but further down, ninth on the list, we find re-imaginings of existing literature. 'There shall be no more novels which are really about other novels. No "modern versions," reworkings, sequels or prequels. No imaginative completions of works left unfinished on their author's death. Instead, every writer is to be issued with a sampler in coloured wools to hang over the fireplace. It reads Knit Your Own Stuff.'

I'd agree with Barnes if works like *Foe* were in fact derivative. But they seem to me instead to be vital additions. And because they rely on inside knowledge, on recognition of the original work, they're like conversations, jokes within the literary family.

I'm not a disinterested party in this. My third novel, *Poe's Cat,* was based on the life and stories of Edgar Allan Poe, which were an echo chamber for my own ideas at the time I was writing, and remain so in the present. Poe, like Beckett, is a writer whose work is closely familiar to me because he wrote about the fluctuations of emotional survival, the way the self fails to wholly stabilise after terrible experiences. The way it can be overwhelmed, as I was after diagnosis, with uncontrollable waves of dread. I'm glad to be free of this – no feeling could be more sickening – but I also want to be reminded of the truth of it, so that I retain an understanding of this part of human experience, a part which may be denied in more stoical or sunnier accounts of survival.

Poe's work is also so fortuitously excessive that it provides a great habitat for the imagination. It's possible to enter a Poe story and settle there, to smile at his extravagance, his breathless murderers, his entranced mourners, his calculating detective Dupin – the predecessor of all literary detectives – and to think.

I enjoy installation art for the same reason, because it includes me within it as a witness, as a living shape that inevitably alters its own architecture. The viewer becomes part of the art, just as the reader of novels is part of the creative process.

Some two hundred kilometres north-west of Kalgoorlie lies the vast saltpan of Lake Ballard, home to an installation by British sculptor Antony Gormley. His *Inside Australia* is a collection of metal figures based on the bodies of local volunteers, who were scanned by laser before a cloth backdrop in the shire hall. Gormley, writing about the transformation of the images that resulted from this, says: 'The process used to find the shape of each sculpture is objective: firstly a twenty second scan, that maps the body in three dimensions with half a million digital co-ordinates. If you then take cross-sections throughout the body, reduce them by two thirds and connect all the contours, you end up with an "Insider". This is a sculpture the same height as the person scanned but one third of the body volume.'

Gormley's description reads like a medical procedure, and brings to mind the work of Wolfgang Laib, the artist who creates floors of pollen which have the capacity to still the mind and entrance the viewer. *Inside Australia* addresses human isolation and transience. On Lake Ballard, a crackled glaze of salt glistens on a surface of red clay. Each figure is placed within view of the others, standing in relaxed grace across ten flat pale kilometres. Not solitary, but not in a defensive cluster. Pathways of footprints run between the sculptures, every impression preserved as if it all happened at the same time: the neat stamp of a wallaby's bound lies next to the bootprints of a man. It's silent, but for the whine of flies and the breath of a slight wind.

The figures stand swaybacked and slightly stooped on their varnish of salt. They have long narrow heads and hold their arms clear of their bodies, so that even though their shapes are abstracted, their postures look human. This is how we hold ourselves when we stand, the neck curving forward just a little from the shoulders. The breasts of the women are like seedpods, angled away from the stalks of the bodies. Thin penises, bulbous and hooked at the tip, jut from the pelvises of the men. Each figure is a durable human shape, unexpected but not pathological, retrieved from a body scan.

My own body, of course, has been scanned many times in order to see what might be going on inside. Within the human body is the whisper of the breath, the heart-music, the voice of the very self: all the things that don't register in machines that have the job of watching out for cancer, all the things that are distinctive to our individual selves. There's something more than biochemical processes and the structures of bones and organs deep inside. Nothing can corrode this inner being, or so we might imagine, in defiance of scientific fact, in our most hopeful art.

The drive from Perth to Lake Ballard takes around ten hours. I enjoy driving; on a long trip I can feel the grain of the road in the wheel under my hands. I like the physical understanding of the distance travelled, the passing vision of bush. But a ten-hour drive alone isn't so pleasant, so I asked Jen, a friend who lives in Melbourne, to come with me.

I first got to know Jen as a child at a beach shack my mother bought in the Yuragir National Park, in northern New South Wales. The shack was on a low cliff at the edge of a small settlement, two streets overlooking a river mouth. It was unlined, weather-beaten, and big enough to accommodate everyone's friends; a refuge for saggy beds, coarse cotton sheets culled from my mother's cupboards, and science-fiction books belonging to my eldest brother – Asimov, Bradbury, Herbert, Heinlen, Philip K. Dick – with cracked spines and cheap, curled-up covers. There was nothing more soothing for me as a child than lying in the hollow of an old mattress, sticky with salt and reading about the Great Nebula, while a high tide rushed in to the cliff-face below.

The land was crowded with wildlife. Western Grey kangaroos with the legs of joeys sticking out of their pouches at all angles observed us from the scrub. Fearless wallabies cropped at dawn just outside the open windows, so that I often woke to the sound of a light snuffling. Goannas with shadowy patterns in their grey hide lifted suddenly from bark or leaf litter, where they had lain invisible. Pythons moved in big loose knots in the branches of banksias. Pelicans circled; sea eagles swerved above the beaches and headlands, watching.

Jen was someone else's friend originally, older than me, but we went walking on bush tracks through the scrub, made sand sculptures, stood on the shore at low tide and worked our bare feet into the sand, catching pipis with our toes. We cooked them over a campfire and ate them, and the bond we created back then still remains.

After driving all morning, we passed through the old gold-mining town of Southern Cross, beyond which the landscape changed. The road ran dead-straight to the horizon, indistinct in the distance. A fire had been through the bush here; eucalypts had puffs of blue-grey growth at the base of blackened trunks. Those trees that weren't marked by fire had dark glossy bark like oiled leather.

I had a strange sense of altitude, of steady flight. In an aeroplane you also move like this, at smooth speed in such a set direction. Jen and I had the music turned up loud in the car – live, lush with applause. Between songs we made plans to go for a walk and have an early dinner once we reached Kalgoorlie, where we would stay the night. We were some fifty kilometres from Coolgardie when we noticed, far in the distance, a figure by the side of the road, the only person we'd seen since Southern Cross.

Closer up, we saw that she was beside a track leading into the bush. She was half crouching, cradling herself. I slowed and pulled over and we hurried from the dusty suburban car that a few moments ago had been like an aeroplane, a pod of happy music, and now sat cooling in the loose gravel. Nothing was moving in the clear bright air, not even the woman, who made no attempt to join us; in fact she stumbled back as we approached. Her clothing was marked with red dirt, and from her responses to Jen's questions we ascertained that she'd been attacked at a picnic area further up the track.

The woman's teeth were clenched; she was barely able to speak. We helped her into the back seat of the car and I drove fast, one hand on the wheel and one reaching back from time to time to touch her ankle in reassurance, as I once did for my son when he too lay on the back seat as I sped down a highway to a hospital. I glanced repeatedly in the rear-vision mirror in case a vehicle from up that track was following, but there was no other traffic on the road. It was as if we three women were alone in the landscape. Even the mobile was out of range.

We reached Coolgardie in under half an hour and drove

straight to the police station, where a policewoman found a quilt for the woman, now stiff with cold as well as pain and fear. She was afraid her attacker might find her, there in the Coolgardie police station, with a tattooed detective at her side.

I had an understanding of the effects of fear: I knew it could stop you in your tracks, I knew it robbed loved objects of meaning, I knew it reduced the hopeful imagination to nothing. I knew, also, that it would pass. But this woman's fear was more extreme than any I'd experienced; even in my times of greatest despair I had been able to speak. I had fought my aggressor metaphorically; this woman had struggled with a physically powerful man. Destruction had taken a human form for her, whereas I had reason to see other people as active in my own defence. She was not, as is a cancer patient, the victim of a biological mistake; someone had made a calculated decision to do her harm.

Moreover there was no clear course of treatment for her. No routine medical procedure, no chemotherapy or radiation, no kind and poetic surgeon. I thought too of the irony of travelling to view sculptures of bodies transformed into metal in an acreage of salt, and unexpectedly having a live body, rigid, silent, agonised, come into our hands.

We were at the police station for five hours, giving statements, waiting for the forensic officer to do her work, sitting with the injured woman, who was eventually able to relax enough to speak. She'd been given clean clothing: dark-blue zippered overalls worn by police to protect crime scenes from contamination. A young policeman told us that he felt helpless and angry, and it helped to hear him say those words. The woman was taken to hospital in Kalgoorlie and we followed, exhausted and uneasy.

In the morning, while Jen slept, I took my cup of tea out to the verandah of our hotel, among the empty junk-food boxes and full ashtrays and crumpled beer cans left by the previous night's drinkers. I stared at the pattern made by the shadow of the iron railing on the floorboards, dazed by the detail of it, over-noticing, dissociating. I couldn't stop my tears.

Yet we were lucky, we three women. I counted the small delays, the hesitations at empty crossroads, the kilometres we travelled at a walking pace behind mining machinery that took up more than one lane on the highway, the stop at the roadhouse where the blade of a knife taken from the cutlery drawer had to be used to open the jammed restroom door. The minutes that passed while that knife was fetched, while it was slotted into the broken lock. The timing that meant Jen and I arrived at the place where the dirt track met the highway just after the woman staggered down to the main road. Every acceleration, every point where I slowed the car, had done the important work of bringing three women together so that one might be saved.

The last town before Lake Ballard is Menzies. From here the road is unsealed, and although it's wide and well maintained its corrugations call for attentive driving. The wheels of earlier travellers had created a track which we tried to follow, but still we swayed and fishtailed in the soft red dust, which clouded the view in the rear-vision mirror.

By mid-morning we were at the lake, walking out onto the glaze of salt, in the footprints of earlier visitors, from one sculptural figure to another. I reminded myself in the silence that all figures exist in relation to one another, that open space is not the same as emptiness, that we reach one another on pathways made by vanished people, that in times of inexplicable destruction, even those caused by human agency, we are still able to be saved.

As we drove back to Kalgoorlie in the early evening, a huge orange moon lifted above the horizon, thin clouds of grey and mauve streaking its surface, and I thought of *Voss*, Patrick White's moon-haunted novel.

Inside Australia could be the subtitle of all White's books, including the one he wrote about himself, *Flaws in the Glass*, and his letters. He could never escape his country. 'How sick I am of the bloody word AUSTRALIA,' he wrote just after the publication of *Voss*, a novel that wasn't universally praised when it first appeared, or even understood. 'What a pity, I am part of it; if I were not, I would get out tomorrow.'

Voss is a love story, but the lovers, Voss and Laura, barely touch. It's a tale of the exploration of a continent, with no great discoveries to report. It's a great wash of imagined and exploratory thought in which Voss, the leader of the expedition, the most strange and intense thinker, is decapitated, his head, at last emptied of thought, thrown across the stony earth.

But this is not a novel about loss and narrowed expectation. Marriage and money, those great preoccupations of the realist novel, don't matter in the world of *Voss*, and nor does public achievement. What matters is the unseen interior of the land and the self, neither of which can ever be settled.

White's Voss is a wayward son, a German medical student who failed to finish his studies because the idea of surgery disgusted him. He is obsessed with the notion of human and geographical interiors as places where he might think and dream. Handling real viscera would contradict everything he values. In any case, Voss is not interested in restoring people to healthy sociability. There are plenty of other men, including his patron Edmund Bonner, concerned with business and community advancement, with the functions and entertainments of the colonial city of Sydney.

Bonner has an orphaned niece, Laura Trevelyan, and the novel opens with a meeting between her and Voss. They seem at first to have little to offer one another: Voss has come to see Bonner, Laura must keep him company until her uncle arrives. Her servant Rose, once a convict, waits on the couple.

The Bonners celebrate the commencement of the expedition with a dinner for the explorer and his ornithologist, the most socially acceptable – in the view of the hostess, Mrs Bonner – of the men who will travel with Voss. When White writes about this dinner he is as brilliant as Virginia Woolf; both are exponents of the swift flicker of sensation, the constant micro-adjustments of human interaction.

White begins his account with a metaphor for possibility: 'That night anything could happen. Two big lamps had transformed the drawing-room into a perfect, luminous egg, which soon contained all the guests.' Laura waits dreamily 'in the solid egg of lamplight, from which they had not yet been born'. Everything is liquid, floating, golden, enclosed.

White is a novelist who writes about details we might notice but don't necessarily remember. The quality of the light. The tiny slippages of connection in a conversation. Everything is volatile, especially between lovers. There is no such thing, in *Voss*, as the conclusive love found in bad romance, that suffocating weight of emotion set like oversweet jelly around living beings.

Laura's thoughts, too, are never still. Over dinner, a guest patronisingly asks what she is thinking and she answers honestly – the pleasure of silence when everyone else is speaking; the sight of quinces, earlier in the evening; garnets, which look like the cooked quinces; poetry; chicken bones and human bones. After the meal, she and Voss bump into one another in the dark garden. Laura smells of chalk and lavender. They tease each other, lapse into seriousness, dissolve a little emotionally, and steady themselves in human isolation.

So much happens in just a few pages, with the characters constantly, lightly, changing their estimation of one another. This is how it is when people first meet and decide to get to know each other. In the garden, outside the yellow lamplight, Laura makes a laughing declaration. 'I am fascinated by you,' she tells Voss. '*You* are *my* desert.' It's an extreme statement, ridiculous, awkward, and true.

Besides the ornithologist, the expedition party includes an ex-convict, a squatter, a strong young English boy, a labourer, a poet and two Aboriginal guides. They represent the types of men who inhabit the colony, each a complicated ambassador of his kind. Their collective task is to traverse the continent from east to west. Voss wants to succeed in this, but he is probably less attracted to the destination than to the very things explorers are supposed to surmount: emptiness and silence.

At the last outpost of European settlement, Voss sends a letter to Laura, a woman he barely knows. He writes formally of his 'great expedition' and 'the many agreeable incidents of the journey thus far'. This sounds conventional and stiff to the modern ear, but for Voss it is a deeply personal letter. He asks two things of Laura. 'My dear Miss Trevelyan, *do not pray for me*, but I would ask you to join me in thought, and exercise of will, daily, hourly, until I may return to you, the victor.' He also asks her to marry him. Or rather, in keeping with the practice of the time, he requests her permission to ask her uncle, Edmund Bonner, for her hand.

The first request invites Laura to form a disembodied connection with Voss, the second is a matter of etiquette and social propriety. Laura, surprised by Voss's letter, writes a thoughtful and honest response. She accepts.

Meanwhile Laura's servant Rose is pregnant. The fact can't be hidden indefinitely, and when it comes to light it preoccupies the Bonner household because it's a conspicuous breach of local ideas of decency. It would be more convenient for the Bonners if Rose or, later, the child, disappeared.

Laura has her own ideas of decency, believing that a mother and baby deserve sanctuary, and Laura grows close to Rose – not in a social sense, but as part of some profound connection with the pregnant woman. Laura, Rose and the unborn baby have a bond that transcends caste and propriety. The women walk in the garden of the mansion in a state of understanding that is close to bliss. When Rose dies soon after giving birth, Laura takes on the role of mother to the child, a scandalous thing to do in her time and place.

During the course of Voss's expedition, Laura is largely occupied with Rose's pregnancy, then with the baby, and with all the conventional activities of a wealthy young woman in the colony, but she also travels, in a dreamy, hallucinatory way, with Voss. And in his final stricken days, Laura falls into a sympathetic agony that cannot be satisfactorily diagnosed. In a way, they have become married; they are one.

But what has happened to Voss? The Aboriginal men, known by their European names of Dugald and Jackie, join the expedition at a station whose owner drinks rum to excess and who props up the leg of a table with the torn-off cover of an edition of Homer. The *Iliad* or the *Odyssey*? White doesn't make this clear. But great tales of voyaging and warfare are reduced to the level of crude domestic expediency in this place, where black women are a sexual convenience and where the European and Aboriginal cultures crumble into joint squalor. When Voss hears the sound of Aboriginal footprints on the earth, he understands that these men own the land, yet he still sees them as his vassals, as subjects who owe him a kind of homage.

The expedition progresses. Christmas is celebrated, there are injuries and illnesses, the country is difficult. Voss writes again to Laura, instructing Dugald to take this letter and others back to the rum drinker's station. But Dugald meets his own people and tears up Voss's letters, which have no significance in his country. He isn't a vassal.

Voss contends with the men's illness, floods, the fatal spearing of the ornithologist. A black man is shot in retaliation. Half the remaining men in the expedition turn back; the ex-convict, the landowner and the labourer have all lost confidence in Voss, who leads the English boy and the poet deeper into the interior. They are compelled to join a group of Aboriginals, where Jackie, their erstwhile guide, changes sides and acts on behalf of his own people.

Voss and his men are dying, in any case, of thirst and starvation. As a comet flares overhead, Voss lies, almost willingly helpless, in a shelter that has been built around them. They are exhausted. The poet destroys his precious notebook filled with visionary writing – which Voss, who has read some of the pages, thinks is a work of madness – and then cuts his own throat. The English boy, too, dies – of starvation and exhaustion.

Voss has a final, enchanted vision of Laura as his wife, riding at his side. Then he is decapitated with his own knife, which he has given to Jackie. Jackie makes hard work of this killing, but eventually an unresisting Voss is cut apart.

Laura knows about the comet, although she is lying sick in bed in the Bonner mansion. Her aunt opens the curtains to reveal the phenomenon, but she refuses to look out. She has already seen it, as part of her strange connection with Voss. Her body is the explorer's companion, physically registering his distant suffering and disintegration. At the moment of his death, she begins her own recovery.

But Laura doesn't fit into colonial society. She's an unmarried woman, the niece – not the daughter – of a rich and important man, the ambiguous mother of a fatherless child. She can't be slighted by the community, and the Bonners love her, but Laura is misplaced. She is not, in her own mind, a marriageable girl and so decides to become a schoolmistress, in violation of her social rank.

Twenty years after the death of Voss, most of the members of the expedition, black and white, are dead. Then the ex-convict, Judd, is discovered living with an inland tribe. His situation is a little like that of the real-life Victorian convict William Buckley, who escaped and survived with tribal people for thirty-two years. (A journalist at the time called Buckley 'Australia's own Robinson Crusoe'.) Back in Sydney, Judd lies wildly about the death of Voss. Laura, who has some deep and physical understanding of Voss's final hours, doesn't dispute his account; she knows too much about Voss to be concerned with Judd's story.

The night sky in *Voss* is eventful. Sometimes, White writes, 'it appeared that men were created only for the hours of darkness', which isn't portrayed as an interruption to labour and progress, but as a place of 'comradeship, dreaming and astronomy'. Voss's journey is moonlit: clouds are described as rags that shine the surface of the moon; the moon is a gravid woman, or a sharp and upright man, or a sea-creature, 'tender, netted' in cloud.

The colonial tasks of mapping and naming, the task of exploration, may falter, the explorer may die, but being dead is less important, White seems to be saying, than being fully alive while you can, being watchful and responsive. Laura, walking among rockpools at a seaside picnic early in the novel, finds vitality and significance in everything: 'In the rapt afternoon all things were all-important, the inquiring mouths of blunt anemones, the twisted roots of driftwood returning and departing in the shallows, mauve scum of little bubbles the sand was sucking down, and the sun, the sun that was hitting them over the heads.' *Voss* is a text of survival because it reveals the constantly shifting glitter of alert consciousness.

The telepathy between Voss and Laura may lie outside our own experience, but we are all capable of the pleasure of sudden sparks of thought, the moments of swift observation with which this novel is charged. At least as important as this is the fact that the reader is invited to consider that we are not isolated in our singular bodies, but rather meet each other, inexplicably, in dreams and thoughts and the delirium of illness.

And in a fundamental sense, we readers are all explorers, until that unimaginable point where all thoughts finish. It isn't distant lovers who speak to us in our ordinary wildernesses – the highway, the office, the hospital room – the disembodied voices that are our invisible companions rise, sometimes lovingly, from the pages of our books. 'One weakens, then it passes, one's strength comes back and one resumes,' says Malone, and he seems, for a moment, to offer this reassurance to me. Both he and the reader know his life is drawing to a close, but there are pages and pages before the end. Thank you, old ruined man, old friend, dreaming in your filthy bed of moons and boats and souls, travelling with me in my mind since I was nineteen.

It's mid-September 2009 but feels like early summer. The acrobatic parrots are breaking off new shoots of the golden robinia that grows on the other side of the courtyard wall. Tucked between the pages of my diary is an appointment card from a clinic where I have my annual check-up for breast cancer. I no longer see the tall surgeon for whom I bought Christmas peonies. The clinic is in the hospital where he first examined me, but is staffed by general practitioners. I don't know the doctor whose name is on the card and I don't mind this; it's good to be in a position where I don't need special attention.

I take the measures that are generally recommended to help avert a recurrence: rarely having alcohol or excess sugar, and avoiding weight gain as best I can, something that's important for survivors of breast cancer because fat retains the oestrogen that promotes the cancer's growth. I no longer push myself into exhaustion, because I cannot recover as quickly as I once did; I am no longer a dictator of my body, to borrow DeLillo's phrase. I swim because it calms me, I wander on the beach because it makes me happy. And on sleepless summer nights, I walk beside the river with my son.

These days I regard my work as not only an occupation but also a confirmation of survival, since storytelling has such an investment in life's continuity. I had always grasped this, of course, but now I understand it with an intense and personal conviction. Increasingly, as time passes, I feel safe, but if my illness were to return, the treatment is at least familiar, and I know how to compose myself, to endure, to ride out the strong emotions. A feeling of dread so powerful it seems like a message of doom is usually just another nightmare, to be remembered once it has passed. All the changes to my life since I was first diagnosed, the good and the bad, have arisen naturally; these are the terms of my daily existence.

On the morning of my appointment, I join the stream of commuter traffic moving from Fremantle into the city. I stop at the Boatshed markets for the newspaper, fresh silverbeet and apples. The check-up will be quick, I tell myself; I can safely leave the food in the car. A famous racing yacht was once built here; now the Boatshed is filled with fruit and flowers, with vegetables, fine cheese, sweet Spanish wafers, all manner of delicious things.

There are boat builders in my family, as well as a wardrobe master. My mother's great-uncles were apprenticed to a shipwright, and their mother was evicted from a hut in northern New South Wales in 1845, in a dispute between two rich men. The matter went to the Privy Council, where one of them was awarded a farthing in damages, or so the story goes. My medical appointment is just another incident in a day that will end well, like all the others. I am one person in a family whose stories lead in many directions.

Back on the highway, I pass the university and follow the river around to the hospital, sitting on its sliver of land between an escarpment and a road. In the car park, attendants are directing traffic. Parking is always difficult at the hospital.

With a few minutes to spare, I sit and gather my thoughts. This is what will happen: I will take the lift to the clinic on the fourth floor. In the waiting room I will read my newspaper – I won't be there long enough for a book. I won't be directed to another floor for a scan, I won't go in and out of a chain of waiting rooms during the course of a day, finishing in the rooms of a surgeon. I won't have an as yet undiscovered cancer. I won't be more than twenty minutes. None of the other people waiting with me will be visibly ill, the very sick will be in the hands of the surgeons and oncologists.

When I'm called into the surgery, when I lie on the examination table, I imagine that the doctor will gaze into the middle distance as she slides her fingers expertly over my skin.

I've taken my anxieties to GPs often enough to know what she will say. She won't tell me that I'm cured, she won't even say that I'm fine. She'll tell me she's speaking only for herself, offering her own informed opinion. She'll say that she can't find anything wrong, and I'll appreciate her honesty. I don't need a written statement assuring my survival. My imagination can work to dampen down fear, make ordinary plans for the future. It can still dream.

'Live and invent,' says poor Malone. In other words, make an honest platform of story in your mind, like a raft, using the sound timber of everything you've loved and read. As with any raft, it may sometimes feel unsteady; it may falter under the weight it must carry, and, over time, it will need repair. It may not withstand the sea for all eternity but nor does it need to – it needs to last a lifespan, nothing more. For the time that it does hold together, you can stand on it like Robinson Crusoe and look back at the site of your own shipwreck, and you can say to yourself, as he did, grateful for being able to say it, 'I am here, not there.'

Sources

PREFACE

Page 3 'You want to give him the book of his own life -', Michael Cunningham, *The Hours*, London, Fourth Estate, 1999, pp. 21–2.

SURGERY

Page 10 'I kiss her cold lips -', quoted in Kenneth Silverman, *Edgar A. Poe: Mournful and Never-ending Remembrance*, New York, HarperCollins, 1992, p. 217.

Page 11 'When poets speak of death -', Ramón Gómez de la Serna, epigraph in Marilyn Yalom, *A History of the Breast*, London, HarperCollins, 1997; 'worked my body hard' (from 'Over the days she worked her body hard') and 'the dictator', Don DeLillo, *The Body Artist*, London, Picador, 2001, p. 57.

Page 12 'there's less charm in life -', Leo Tolstoy, *Anna Karenina*, trans. Constance Garnett, New York, Barnes and Noble, 2003, p. 351.

Page 15 'Sunset and evening star -', Alfred Tennyson, in *Tennyson's Poetry*, ed. Robert W. Hill, New York, J.R. Norton, 1971, p. 496.

Page 16 details about Samuel Beckett and *The Divine Comedy* come from James Knowlson, *Damned to Fame: The Life of Samuel Beckett*, Bloomsbury, London, 1997, p. 53.

Page 21 ' "I have been fashioned -', Vladimir Nabokov, *Invitation to a Beheading*, London, Penguin, 2001, p. 20.

Page 22 Ann and Reg Cartwright, *Norah's Ark*, London, Random House, 1983.

Page 24 'uphill work', and page 25: 'I felt as if he had -', Charles Dickens, *Bleak House*, London, Penguin, 1971, p. 285, 680.

Page 31 'The pleasantest of all diversions -', Yoshida Kenko, *Essays in Idleness*, trans. Donald Keene, New York, Columbia University Press, 1967, p. 12.

Page 32 'Thus he spoke in memory -', Ki No Tsurayuki, *The Tosa Diary*, trans. William N. Porter, Vermont, Charles E. Tuttle & Co, 1981, pp. 97–8, 133.
Page 33 'a wonderful physical -' and 'if we could answer their love -', E.M. Forster, *Where Angels Fear to Tread*, Harmondsworth, Penguin, 1975, p. 125.
Page 34 'I have made you -', Isaiah, 46:4.
Page 40 'Praise life while you walk -' David Campbell, 'The Return of the Captain', *Hardening of the Light: Selected Poems*, Ginninderra, Ginninderra Press, 2006, p. 79.
Page 41 'Live and invent', Samuel Beckett, *The Beckett Trilogy: Molloy, Malone Dies, The Unnamable*, London, Picador, 1976, p. 179; 'I am a great believer -', Saul Bellow, *Ravelstein*, London, Penguin, 2000, p. 231.
Page 44 'For Colette, *Les Misérables* -', Alberto Manguel, *A History of Reading*, London, HarperCollins, 1997, p. 151; 'soul denied in vain -', Samuel Beckett, op. cit., p. 204; Don DeLillo, *Falling Man*, London, Picador 2008, p. 234.
Page 45 'Can I not everywhere -', Dante Alighieri, *The Divine Comedy*, trans. & introduced by Kenneth Mackenzie, London, The Folio Society, 1979, p. xv.
Page 47 details about the life of Samuel Beckett come from James Knowlson, op. cit.; 'A little darkness, in itself -', Samuel Beckett, op. cit., p.203.
Page 48 'He scooped his fingers -', Samuel Beckett, *More Pricks than Kicks*, London, Picador, 1974, p. 9.

CHEMOTHERAPY

Page 57 'I feel thick-headed -', Joyce Wadler, *My Breast: One Woman's Cancer Story*, Reading MA, Addison Wesley, 1992, p. 162.
Page 58 'He stared out of the window -', Alan Hollinghurst, *The Line of Beauty*, London, Picador, 2004, p. 411.
Page 61 'He did not believe -', Leo Tolstoy, op. cit., p. 484.
Page 63 Martin Amis, 'What happened to Me on Holiday', in *Heavy Water and Other Stories*, London, Jonathan Cape, 1998.

Page 69 details of H.G. Wells' funeral come from Paul Johnson, 'And Another Thing', *The Spectator*, 3 May 2008.
Page 73 'the soul's stutter', James Wood, *The Irresponsible Self: On Laughter and the Novel*, New York, Picador, 2005 pp. 33, 219.
Page 76 'had to fight back an uneasy desire ~', quoted in Tom Griffiths, 'Flying Fox and Drifting Sand: Going with the Flow', in *Storykeepers*, ed. Marion Halligan, Sydney, Duffy and Snellgrove, 2001, p. 150.
Page 77 'True! – nervous – very ~', Edgar Allan Poe, 'The Tell-Tale Heart' in *The Complete Tales and Poems of Edgar Allan Poe*, London, Penguin, 1982, p. 303.
Page 78 'made us remember at least ~', quoted in Douglas Kahn, *Noise Water Meat: A History of Sound in the Arts*, Cambridge, Massachusetts, MIT Press, 2001, p. 66.
Page 79 'the deaf do not, because they cannot ~', David Wright, *Deafness: A Personal Account*, London, Allen Lane, 1969, p. 81; 'Silent men, moving unheard ~', Joseph Conrad, *Under Western Eyes*, Edinburgh, John Grant, 1925, p. 369.
Page 81 'one mustn't underestimate ~', Donna Tartt, *The Secret History*, Ringwood, Penguin, 2008, p. 182.
Page 82 'White sky ~', 'The objects in the room ~', 'I lay on my bed ~' and 'if one is to read Dante ~', ibid., p. 422, 276, 551–2, 184.
Page 87 anecdote about Saul Bellow is from Philip Roth, 'I Gotta Scheme: The Words of Saul Bellow', *The New Yorker*, 25 April 2005, p. 74.
Page 88 'By a curious irony ~' and 'I seem to spend ~', quoted in Susan Sontag, *Illness as Metaphor and Aids and its Metaphors*, New York, Picador 1988, p. 33.
Page 89 'out of this nettle ~', quoted by Dymphna Cusack in a letter to Florence James, in *Yarn Spinners: A Story in Letters*, ed. Marilla North, St Lucia, University of Queensland Press, 2001, p. 16.
Page 93 'I had a dream once ~', Marilynne Robinson, *Gilead*, London, Virago, 2005, pp. 230–1.

RADIATION

Page 98 'he went on to explain -', John Hersey, *Hiroshima*, London, Hamish Hamilton, 1966, p. 88.

Page 101 'That is what people do -,' David Hare, screenplay of *The Hours*, produced by Scott Rudin, directed by Stephen Daldry.

Page 103 'not out of sentimentality -' and 'The warmth, the smell -', Viktor Shklovsky, *Zoo or Letters not about Love*, trans. & ed. Richard Sheldon, Ithaca, Cornell University Press, 1971, pp. 87, 31.

Page 105 'Here in the dockyard -', Aage Utzon, in Geraldine Brooks, 'Unfinished Business: Jørn Utzon Returns to the Opera House', *The New Yorker*, 17 October 2005, p. 100.

Page 106 'I should still recommend -', Vladimir Nabokov, *Lectures on Literature*, San Diego, Harcourt, 1980, p. 371.

Page 107 'This whole plot -', Paul Theroux, 'The Best Year of My Life', *The New Yorker*, 14 November 2005, p. 89.

Page 109 'that must prevent them -', quoted in Roger Nichols, *Debussy Remembered*, London, Faber, 1992, p.37.

Page 110 detail on Murasaki and the writing of *The Tale of Genji* is from William J. Puette, *A Reader's Guide: The Tale of Genji*, Boston, Tuttle, 1983, and Ivan Morris, *The World of the Shining Prince: Court Life in Ancient Japan*, New York, Kodansha, 1994.

Page 111 'One can visit a spot -', Murasaki Shikibu, *The Tale of Genji*, trans. & introduced by Edward G. Seidensticker, New York, Alfred A. Knopf, 1992, p. vii.

Page 113 'I was extremely lucky -', Royall Tyler, 'Genji the Proud', address to the Genji Millenium Committee. (Text of this lecture kindly supplied to the author; my reading of *The Tale of Genji* rests on the account of the novel in this address.)

Page 121 'a boat upon the waters', William J. Puette, op. cit. p. 172; 'there's a story for you -', Samuel Beckett, op. cit., p. 374.

Page 122 'In the midst of life's fullness ~', Walter Benjamin, *Illuminations*, trans. Harry Zohn, New York, Schocken, 1969, p.87; 'Think of it this way ~', Haruki Murakami, 'The Novelist in Wartime,' http://www.salon.com/books/feature/2009/02/20/haruki_murakami/index.html.

Page 123 'in art you become familiar ~', Saul Bellow, *Ravelstein*, London, Penguin, 2000, p. 47.

Page 126 'The hard lump of his tumour ~', Aleksandr Solzhenitsyn, *Cancer Ward*, New York, Farrar Straus and Giroux, 1991, p. 10.

Page 127 'Yefrem just did not feel ~', ibid., p. 103.

Page 128 'These literary tragedies ~' and 'like a drug', 'a blessing', ibid., pp. 482, 481.

Page 130 'I shall go on in the same way ~', Leo Tolstoy, op. cit., p. 754.

Page 132 'It is at the heart of my moral code ~', Barack Obama, *The Audacity of Hope*, Edinburgh, Canongate, 2007, p. 66; Alex Miller, *Landscape of Farewell*, Crows Nest, Allen & Unwin, 2007.

Page 133 'he compares the process ~', Timothy W. Ryback, *Hitler's Private Library*, New York, Alfred A. Knopf, 2008 pp. 115, 209.

RECONSTRUCTION

Page 140 'as though she had been born ~' and 'gladdened her feet', Leo Tolstoy, op. cit., p. 73; 'the right coat, the right dress ~', Linda Grant, *The Thoughtful Dresser*, London, Virago, 2009, p. 300.

Page 141 Linda Grant, ibid.

Page 142 'When she put on a white blouse ~', Jonathan Franzen, *The Corrections*, London, Harper Perennial, 2007, pp. 502–3.

Page 143 'the means by which you ~', Linda Grant, op. cit., p. 13.

Page 145 'We are born reading ~', William S. Wilson, 'Loving/Reading', in *Antaeus: Literature as Pleasure*, ed. Daniel Halperin, London, Collins Harvill, 1990, pp. 200–201; 'there is nothing more ~', J.M. Coetzee, *Elizabeth Costello*, Sydney, Knopf, 2003, p. 150.

Page 151 'I got in over my head -', quoted in Carolyn Burke, *Lee Miller on Both Sides of the Camera*, London, Bloomsbury, 2006, p.367.

Page 152 'we are a wonderful people -', Edgar Allan Poe, 'The Man that Was Used Up', *The Complete Tales and Poems of Edgar Allan Poe*, London, Penguin, 1982, p. 407; 'war is beautiful -', quoted in Walter Benjamin, Illuminations: Essays and Reflections, New York, Schocken, 1969, p. 241.

Page 153 'prodigies of valor', Edgar Allan Poe, op. cit., Penguin, 1982, pp. 407–408.

Page 154 'man that is born of a woman -', Edgar Allan Poe, ibid., p. 408; 'Many people everywhere -', Donald Ritchie, *A Tractate on Japanese Aesthetics*, Berkeley, Stone Press Bridge, 2007, p. 38.

Page 156 'I'll be happy if you' and 'My heart seems to be -', dialogue from *Tokyo Story*, feature film directed by Yasujiro Ozu, 1953.

Page 157 'Japanese ghosts have -', Junichiro Tanizaki, *In Praise of Shadows*, Stony Creek, Leete's Island Books, 1977, p. 30.

Page 159 'meat', 'I was worried about her -' and 'People think that -', Philip Roth, *The Dying Animal*, London, Vintage, 2002, pp. 2, 40, 99–100.

Page 160 'The marriage of true minds -', Saul Bellow, *Ravelstein*, London, Penguin, 2000, p. 120.

Page 161 'heroic optimism' and 'hands are cut off -', Marina Warner, *From the Beast to the Blonde*, London, Vintage, 1994, pp. xvi, xv.

Page 165 George Prochnik, 'The Porcupine Illusion,' *Cabinet Magazine Online*, Issue 26 Summer 2007.

Page 167 'in the depths of the sea -' and 'Take into the air -', Samuel Beckett, 'Belaqua and the Lobster' in *More Pricks than Kicks*, London, Picador, 1974, p. 19.

Page 168 'She began telling me -', Philip Roth, op. cit., p. 129.

Page 169 'There is nothing for which you -', quoted in Parmenia Migel, *Titania: The Biography of Isak Dinesen*, London, Michael Joseph, 1967, p.111.

Page 170 'Now she felt, with horror –' and 'strange warfare', Isak Dinesen, *Winter's Tales,* Harmonsworth, Penguin, 1983, pp. 38, 41.
Page 172 'pearls are like poet's tales –', Isak Dinesen, *Anecdotes of Destiny*, London, University of Chicago Press, 1958, p. 12.
Page 173 the idea of narration holding the promise of staying alive comes from Jane Smiley, *Thirteen Ways of Looking at the Novel*, New York, Reading MA, Anchor Books, 2006, p. 100.

SURVIVAL

Page 179 details of factors that predispose women to breast cancer are from a study in *New England Journal of Medicine*, 14 October 2004, cited in *Keeping Abreast: A Quarterly Newsletter about Breast Cancer Research*, produced by Dr David Ingram, December 2004, p. 9.
Page 183 'Sometimes I sit with one of them –', Erich Maria Remarque, *All Quiet on the Western Front*, trans. Brian Murdoch, London, Vintage 1996, p. 121.
Page 184 'My hands are lying –', ibid., p. 122.
Page 185 'devour' and 'the war will sink –', ibid., p. 123.
Page 187 details of the Japanese campaign in Papua New Guinea are from Paul Ham, *Kokoda*, Sydney, HarperCollins, 2005, pp. 517–18.
Page 188 'when they realised the full significance –', Paul Ham, ibid., p. 515.
Page 190 'I thought I might say to him –', Roy Hutcheson Campbell, Andrew S. Skinner, *Adam Smith*, London, Croom Helm, 1985, p. 188.
Page 191 'By Allah I will not –', T*he Book of a Thousand Nights and a Night*, trans. Richard F. Burton, privately printed by the Burton Club, p. 29.
Page 192 'certain books are so prodigally –', J.M. Coetzee, *Elizabeth Costello*, Sydney, Knopf, 2003, pp. 13, 14; 'I think of you as –', J.M. Coetzee, *Foe*, Penguin, 1988, p. 50.
Page 193 'There I lay sprawled –', ibid., p. 5.
Page 194 'knows above all how many –', ibid., p. 94.

Page 195 'Is it better to be -', Daniel Defoe, *Robinson Crusoe*, London, Penguin, 1988, p. 80.

Page 197 details of medical studies of cancer treatment are from Susan M. Love's afterword to Joyce Wadler, op. cit., p.179.

Page 199 'inventory' Samuel Beckett, *The Beckett Trilogy*, op. cit., p. 167; 'There shall be no more novels -', Julian Barnes, *Flaubert's Parrot*, London, Picador, 1984, p. 99.

Page 201 'The process used to find -', Antony Gormley, 'Inside Australia' (booklet), Perth International Arts Festival, 2003, p. 2.

Page 208 'How sick I am -', Patrick White, in *Patrick White: Letters*, ed. David Marr, Sydney, Random House, 1994, p. 130.

Page 210 'That night anything could -', Patrick White, *Voss*, London, Vintage, 1994, p. 80.

Page 211 'I am fascinated -', 'great expedition' and 'the many agreeable -', ibid., pp. 88, 153.

Page 215 'Australia's own Robinson Crusoe', John Morgan, quoted in Barry Hill, 'Buckley, Our Imagination, Hope', in Robyn Gardner, ed., *Writings on the Shipwreck Coast*, Port Fairy, Mattoid/Grange, 2008, p. 36; 'it appeared that men -', 'comradeship, dreaming -', 'tender, netted' and 'In the rapt afternoon -', Patrick White, *Voss*, op. cit., pp. 376, 359, 286, 62.

Page 216 'One weakens, then it passes -', Samuel Beckett, *The Beckett Trilogy*, op. cit., p. 231.

Acknowledgements

I would like to thank my publisher Ben Ball, who encouraged me to write this book and offered welcome latitude and direction, Meredith Rose for her fine and thoughtful editing, and Peter Straus for representing my work.

I'd also like to thank all those who provided useful responses to *Reading by Moonlight* at various stages: James Bradley for listening as the idea for the book formed, Delia Falconer for literary and general clarity, Deborah Robertson and Sarah Hay for many helpful suggestions, John Scott for instructing me on the finer points of Dante's moon-viewing, Royall Tyler for his generous communications, Alex Miller for conversations about stories and empathy, John Kaldor for liking the tower and correcting my description of the processes of cancer, Michael Levine for alerting me to Schopenhauer's porcupines, Philip Mead for reading my account of *Voss*, Jen Jewell Brown for travelling with me, Mark Ramsey and Anita Ramsey for reading an early version, Shirley Walker for sound advice always, and my son Tom. I would also like to thank Sister Rita Goodchild for permission to use her story.

Certain names in the text have been changed where friends prefer to retain their anonymity.

Some sections of this book have been previously published, in an earlier form, as 'The Peonies' in *Thanks for the Mammaries*, ed. Sarah Darmody, Camberwell, Penguin, 2009; 'The Long Fall into Steel' in *The Best Australian Essays 2005*, ed. Robert Dessaix, Melbourne, Black Inc., 2005; 'Over Mountains and Black Water' in *Daughters and Fathers*, ed. Carmel Bird, St Lucia, University of Queensland Press, 1997; 'Big Animals' in *The Best Australian Stories 2008*, ed. Delia Falconer, Melbourne, Black Inc., 2008; 'Burning Down the House' in *The Bulletin*, Summer Reading Edition, December 2006.